SUCCESSFUL STRESS CONTROL

Looks at what stress is, at what it does—good and bad—
and at ways to alleviate the effects of stress,
principally with herbal remedies

By the same author:

The Herb User's Guide
The Holistic Herbal
Welsh Herbal Remedies

Successful Stress Control

THE NATURAL WAY

David Hoffmann

THORSONS PUBLISHERS, INC.
Rochester, Vermont
Wellingborough, Northamptonshire

Thorsons Publishers, Inc.
One Park Street
Rochester, Vermont 05767

First U.S. edition 1987

Library of Congress Cataloging in Publication Data

Hoffmann, David, 1951–
  Successful stress control.

  Bibliography: p.
  Includes index.
  1. Stress (Psychology) 2. Therapeutics,
Physiological. I. Title. [DNLM: 1. Stress—
popular works. 2. Stress, Psychological—
prevention & control—popular works. WM 172 H711s]
BF575.S75H63   1987   158'.1   86-30110
ISBN 0-7225-1051-9 (pbk.)

Printed and bound in the United States

10 9 8 7 6 5 4 3 2 1

Distributed to the book trade in the
United States by Harper and Row

Distributed to the book trade in Canada by Book Center, Inc.,
Montreal, Quebec

Distributed to the health food trade in Canada by Alive Books,
Toronto and Vancouver

Contents

SUCCESSFUL STRESS CONTROL

ONE

Wholeness and Healing

Stress, anxiety, and tension seem to be common characteristics of our lives today. Change is in the air. It is the keynote of all we see, do, and hear. Our lives are being transformed from within and without, painlessly changing at times and painfully changing at others, but always in flux. The skills demanded by our jobs are shifting, as are the goals and expectations of society itself. Nothing seems to have a solid foundation, whether it be family relationships, the workplace, the national economy, or international politics. It's almost as if society is going through its adolescence! It is a time of chaos and crisis, a time of great stress, and yet a time of great opportunity.

In this book, we'll look at what stress is, at what it does – both good and bad – and at how to remove the weight it lays on our shoulders. There are many techniques that can help and we shall look at a few of them, focusing particularly on the use of herbs. However, bear in mind that to relieve stress, anxiety, and tension in any truly meaningful way also involves finding one's own healing heart – our center of stillness and peace in this all-embracing environment of change. Some of us call this center God, others call it our Essential Humanity. What we call it is unimportant; the important thing is that we experience it as real and vital.

If we are to come to terms with stress rather than be slaves to its dictates, we must give some thought to what we want as a positive alternative. To be truly free of stress, we would have to be truly free. Whether we attain this rare and enviable state or not, we can all work toward being whole within ourselves, since it is this wholeness that is the basis for ease, which is the opposite of stress. In these times of confusion, ease does not enter our lives by default. We must create an environment of wholeness and then invite it in.

When we are feeling "stressed out," we are in fact experiencing ourselves as un-whole. One interpretation of the psychological imbalance that characterizes our society is that, consciously or unconsciously, we are experiencing a deep sense of separation, of alienation, from our roots. Every parent knows the anguish of children separated from their fathers or mothers. What we in the "civilized" West have done, without realizing it, is to alienate ourselves from our spiritual mother, Mother Earth. No wonder that our modern scourges are stress and fear. We have lost our roots.

THE ROLE OF HERBS

The use of herbs in the healing process reestablishes our connection with our roots, thereby promoting the sense of wholeness that is essential to successful healing and feelings of ease. Herbalism is based on relationships – between plant and person, between plant and planet, and hence between person and planet. Using herbs in the healing process means taking part in an ecological cycle. This offers us the opportunity to be consciously involved in the living, vital world of which we are part. Herbs can link us into the broader context of planetary wholeness, so that while they are doing their healing job, we can do ours. To create an environment of wholeness and invite ease into our lives, our job is to be aware of the remedies we use and of the links and relationships we establish with our world by using them.

As an example, let's consider the treatment of a stomach ulcer, first with drugs and then with herbs. With drug treatment, problems arise immediately. One of the drugs frequently used for illnesses related to over-production of stomach acid is Tagamet. This medication works by rapidly changing some of the biochemistry that leads to ulcer formation and irritation, reducing discomfort and making life more bearable. However, in the broader context, Tagamet raises a moral dilemma. The chemical process used to make this drug is renowned for the pollution it produces. So instead of linking those who take it with nature's wholeness, it creates an immediate relationship with nature's pain, a direct relationship between their stomachs and dead fish in a polluted river. Consider also the laboratory animals that died in the development of the drug, and the dependence on a multinational pharmaceutical industry not well known for its selfless service!

Contrast these results with using herbal remedies to treat the same condition. Comfrey, marshmallow root, meadowsweet, and golden seal can all be used to soothe and heal an ulcer. The pain and discomfort go away and, with the right diet and life style, the ulcer heals and need not come back. However, herbal remedies also offer us the chance to become aware of the way in which the environment (through plants) is actively healing us. By attuning ourselves to the plants and their healing qualities, we establish a rapport with nature. In this way, the treatment of the ulcer becomes part of a deeper transformation process.

We can only truly ease our stress-related "dis-eases," such as ulcers, if we acknowledge the social and cultural context in which the disease and the desired healing take place. It is a therapeutic and moral mistake to use herbal remedies to relieve our physical and psychological distress if we are going to return to our usual alienated lives and continue in patterns of thought, behavior, work, and culture that are themselves the source of the disease. We are at home on this planet – we have only to recognize it. Through their power to alleviate the very ills of humanity, herbal remedies provide a clue, a signpost, to this reality: We are part of a wonderfully integrated whole. This is not the stuff of vague idealism or mysticism but an essential truth that is the basis for this book and for the whole of herbal medicine.

TWO

What Is Stress?

There are several ways to define stress. Perhaps the most encompassing is: "Stress is the response of the body to any demand." Just staying alive creates demands on the body for life-maintaining energy; even while we are asleep, our bodies continue to function. So by this definition, stress is a fundamental part of being alive and should not be avoided! The trick is to ensure that the degree of stress we experience is such that life is a joy, not a drag.

From this perspective, energy usage is one characteristic of stress. Another characteristic is lack of specificity. Any demands made upon us in daily life bring about certain reactions in the body. These same reactions occur under a whole range of different conditions, both physical and emotional – from hot and cold to joy and sorrow. As aware, feeling people, we probably make a big distinction between the pain caused by the loss of a loved one and the pain caused by the temperature dropping too fast; but the nature of the demand is unimportant at the biological level. To the body, it's all the same because the stress response is always the same. Nerve signals are sent from the brain to several glands, and these react by secreting hormones to cope with the task ahead. So stress is not just worry and strain. It is a keynote of life, with all its ups and downs. A new and exciting love can cause us as much stress as an old and cranky boss!

The range of responses triggered by stress demonstrates the intricate ties that exist between the mental and physical components of who we are. Before we look a little closer at these responses, it may be useful to review some of the scientific theories about stress. It may seem that many of these theories revolve around minor semantic differences. I'm afraid that appears to be the level of the research on the topic to date. Bear with me for a while!

SCIENTIFIC THEORIES

Theories about stress tend to fall into three categories:

1. Stress as a stimulus: this category attempts to describe the various unpleasant situations that cause stress.

2. Stress as a response: this category attempts to describe the responses that occur in the body or the mind when we are confronted by an unpleasant situation.

3. Stress as a perceived threat: this category views stress as a reflection of our own perception that we cannot cope with our environment.

Let's look at each of these in turn.

Stress as a Stimulus

Stimulus-based approaches to stress are concerned with identifying aspects of the environment that have an unpleasant effect on us. This very simple approach views human stress as being the same as the physical stress involved in an engineering project like building a bridge. The concern is with identifying stressful situations and determining how and why they affect the mind and body. This category of research has focused mostly on the workplace and on factors such as ambient noise levels and heat, as well as things like job demands. Working under deadlines with large amounts of information to be processed would be rated as stressful under this approach, as would be monotony, isolation, and situations in which we have little control over events.

Viewing stress this way is fine if we think of people as girder bridges, but that's not how an herbalist views them! Two of the problems with this mechanistic approach to stress are:

1. Particular situations are not inherently stressful, and there is a large variation in their effect on different people. For example, the noise of a disco is stressful for some people, while others thrive on it.

2. There are even variations in the same individual's responses to the same situation at different times. Whether we are well rested or fatigued might determine how stressful we find traffic jams, for example.

It seems difficult to define a situation as stressful without taking into account the responses of the people who might be involved. The degree of stress a particular environment might cause has to be seen as a spectrum. There is no doubt that, for most people, walking down the meridian of a freeway to look for a gas station would be stressful, while watching a sunset from a flower-strewn mountain meadow would have little inherent stress, unless it's June and you have hayfever!

Stress as a Response

The second category of physiological theory we'll look at views stress as the response to an adverse, or stressful, situation. This approach is based on the work of the physiologist Hans Selye. Selye theorized that the stress response is a built-in mechanism that comes into play whenever demands are placed on us, and is therefore a defense reaction with a protective and adaptive function. In other words, there is a general physiological reaction to all forms of stress, which usually acts in our own best interests. Selye called this reaction the general adaptation syndrome (GAS).

This theory suggests a three-stage process of response:

1. An alarm reaction.

2. A resistance stage, which represents a functional recovery of the body to a level superior to the pre-stress state.

3. An exhaustion reaction, in which there is a depletion and breakdown of the recovery of stage 2, due to continuation of the stressful situation.

The limitation of this inflexible physiological model of stress is that it ignores the purely emotional or mental factors that can produce a wide variation in the way we respond to potentially stressful situations.

Stress as a Perceived Threat

Much recent research suggests that specific situations or objects are threatening to us because we perceive them as such, rather than because of any inherent characteristics. According to this category of research, stress occurs when we cannot cope with or adjust to the demands made on us – when it all becomes too much. The degree of stress is partially affected by what is going on in general, but is more intimately connected with how we perceive the factors involved and how we are feeling at the time.

RESPONSES TO STRESS

There is now a large body of research about both the physiological and the psychological responses to stress. It is easier to explore these responses separately, as we'll do here, but keep in mind that they need to be looked at in conjunction with each other in order to be fully understood.

Physiological Responses

The regulation of physiological responses to threats or stressful demands is handled mainly by the adrenal gland. Immediate response is controlled mainly, though not completely, by the adrenal gland's central medulla, while long-term response is handled by the surrounding cortex.

The initial response – preparing the body for what has been called the fight-or-flight reaction – involves:

1. Increased nervous-system activity.

2. Release of adrenalin and/or noradrenalin into the blood stream by the adrenal medulla. These hormones support the nervous system through metabolic activity. The body's response to these chemicals includes:

a. increase in heart rate and blood pressure.

b. surface constriction of blood vessels, so that the blood leaves the skin to provide the muscles with more sugar and oxygen (which is why we go white with shock).

c. mobilization of the liver's energy reserves through the release of stored glucose.

If the stressful situation is very intense or continues over a period of time, the adrenal cortex becomes increasingly involved in the stress reaction. The activity of the cortex is largely controlled by blood levels of adrenocorticotrophic hormone (ACTH), which is released by the anterior pituitary gland. When information about sustained stress has been "processed" by the central nervous system, a whole range of new bodily responses occurs, and it is these longer-term reactions that can adversely affect the quality of life.

Psychological Responses

In general terms, the psychological reaction to stress takes the following course:

1. The initial fight-or-flight reaction is accompanied by emotions such as anxiety or fear.

2. Individual ways of coping are activated as we attempt to find a way of dealing with the harmful or unpleasant situation.

3. If the coping strategies are successful, the fight-or-flight reaction and the anxiety state subside.

4. If the coping strategies fail and the stress situation continues, a range of psychological reactions, including depression and withdrawal, may occur.

The implication is that the consequences of failing to cope can be serious, and it is therefore important that we develop our own ways of adapting to and successfully dealing with stressful situations.

Research about how we cope has defined two broad categories of coping strategies. The first involves attempts to change our unsatisfactory relationship with the environment. Examples of this category would be:

1. Escaping from the unpleasant situation – not always possible!

2. Preparing ourselves for situations that we anticipate will be stressful. This might involve thinking ahead of time about the situation and its likely impact, thereby preparing ourselves adequately for the event; or it might involve some actual work – for example, studying for an exam, instead of just worrying about it.

The second category of response research involves "palliative" strategies that attempt to soften the impact of the stress once it has occurred. Examples of this category include:

1. Denial, by which we refuse to acknowledge all or some of the threat in the situation.

2. Intellectualization, by which we detach ourselves emotionally from the situation.

Both of these strategies serve to protect us and help us maintain a reasonable equilibrium through difficult times, but there is always the danger that such strategies may make it more difficult for us to resolve a problem and may become established as part of our psychological makeup.

Other coping strategies, including various relaxation techniques, may be appropriate in some or all cases. However, the use of such strategies may delay the direct reaction that we need to solve the problem that is causing the stress. This is also true of another, particularly destructive way of coping: escaping via the use of alcohol, tranquilizers, or other drugs.

There are some stresses for which no clear solution exists – for example, caring for the chronically ill – and in such situations softening the impact of stress may be the only way for us to cope.

If stress is long-term or particularly severe, marked emotional changes may take place. If the coping strategies we employ don't work, we may regard the situation as one for which there is no solution and increasingly see ourselves as unable to control the events of our lives. Hopelessness and helplessness are both likely to give rise to feelings of depression, and may even lead to suicidal thoughts. Following the stress of chronic illness, for example, patients may literally give up hope. If this occurs, they may become not only emotionally disturbed but also more vulnerable to further physical illness.

Factors Affecting Our Responses

Although we can talk in general terms about physiological and psychological response patterns, we should remember that these patterns are by no means fixed. For each one of us, the pattern of response to stress is determined by many factors, some of which are listed below.

Previous experience

Once we have experienced a particular stressful situation, we are usually able to cope better with it if it comes up again. The experience provides us with knowledge about the situation and puts us in a more predictable position. We are more aware of how our behavior will affect a potentially stressful environment and how we will be affected by it. For example, the second visit to a doctor is usually easier than the first.

Information

Information about an impending stressful event allows us to make preparations that will ease the impact and intensity of our reactions to the stress. It is well known, for example, that describing surgical procedures and typical post-operative reactions, including pain, to patients can often aid recovery. However, personality differences must be taken into account. People differ radically in their response to the stresses associated with illness.

Individual differences

Some people try to protect themselves from the full impact of the stress by denying, playing down, or emotionally detaching themselves from the situation. Providing information to these people may actually increase their stress levels, rather than decreasing them.

Social support

Not surprisingly, the impact of stressful events is affected by our social systems. Support and empathy from others greatly softens the degree of reaction to stress, especially when we are young and our patterns of behavior, response, and perception are developing. It seems that insufficient early social support can give rise to physical and behavioral problems, including a reduced ability to withstand stress.

Response to stress can be eased by support from either the family or the community. For example, the recovery of patients from strokes can be significantly affected by the understanding and empathy shown by their families or friends, and studies have shown that women who have close, confiding relationships are less likely to develop stress-related psychiatric problems. It is not surprising, then, that the loss of a close relationship, which represents a sudden and severe loss of support, is rated among the most stressful of all life events.

It says a lot about our rational and analytical approach to life that research is needed in order for the medical profession to acknowledge that caring and support are vital parts of the healing process. Our humanity should tell us that!

Control

The degree to which we believe we can control a situation has an important impact on the degree to which that situation is likely to cause us stress. Research has shown that the most harmful and distressing situations are those in which we feel entirely helpless, believing that nothing we can do will significantly alter the outcome. This is a good reason to take power and information away from the "experts" and put it in the hands of people like you and me, thereby restoring our sense of control. It is also the reason why this book focuses on herbs and other stress-fighting allies that we can use ourselves, rather than relying on the diagnostic powers and prescriptions of others.

The need to take back responsibility for our own well being becomes acute when we realize that the tremendous progress made in the medical sciences in recent years has not brought with it any significant improvement in our overall health. In fact, the incidence of some diseases is on the increase. Heart problems, digestive maladies, and mental disturbances are striking people in their thirties, forties, and fifties. The underlying cause of many of the diseases that are common today is undoubtedly stress.

It is true that great strides have been made toward the control of infectious diseases, and medical research has increased our understanding of disease processes. But too much attention has been given to treatment after the fact – to intervention and cure rather than to prevention. With the cost of treatment and hence the cost of health insurance soaring, we would do well to find out as much as we can about the causes of the diseases that afflict us, and to use any means at our disposal to forestall their development. It is therefore worth spending some time here to consider in greater depth the relationship between stress and illness.

STRESS AND ILLNESS

Statistical studies have shown a clear association between increased incidence of disease and the presence of one or more of the factors discussed below.

Social Class

Many of the common fatal illnesses tend to occur with higher incidence in the "lower" social classes. The reasons for this are not fully understood, but probably revolve around such factors as diet, housing conditions, employment/unemployment, and quality of medical care. In addition, a feeling of security – financial and otherwise – is basic to any sense of well being. A sense of personal power and control over one's own life are as important to our health as is a good diet.

Occupation

Some types of work, as well as the physical and social attributes of the work environment, are associated with higher levels of physiological and psychological illness. The factors known to be involved include:

1. Shift work, because of the disruption of circadian rhythms and social life.

2. Long hours (75 hours per week or more).

3. Physically adverse conditions, such as cramped or noisy quarters and bad lighting.

4. Changes in work environment, such as to a different line of work or level of responsibility. Significantly more heart attacks occur in the year following such changes.

5. Boring, repetitive work, which can produce increases in frequency of depression, sleep disturbances, and stomach disorders.

6. Responsibility and deadline pressures, which can result in a higher risk of conditions such as high blood pressure and ulcers.

Remember that not all people react adversely to these conditions. Many people cope quite well with demanding work environments, and may even appear to thrive in them. As I've said before, jobs are not inherently stressful; rather it is when we have difficulty in coping with the demands, changes, or monotony of a certain job that the job becomes unpleasant and increases the risk of ill health.

Unemployment can also lead to higher risk of illness, brought about by a major life change and possible loss of self-esteem. Work meets not only financial but also social and psychological needs, and failure to meet those needs carries a high personal cost in terms of mental and physical well being.

Life Style

A lot of research has centered around identifying two basic life styles, known as type A and type B. The type A personality is competitive, striving, and usually under pressure; type B is more relaxed and calm. Type A exhibits what has been called the coronary-prone behavior pattern, because of increased chances of coronary heart disease. Other life styles supposedly represent various combinations of type A and type B, with proportional degrees of stress and propensity toward stress-induced diseases. The impact of different life styles will be explored in greater depth later, in the section on heart disease.

Life Events

A number of studies have demonstrated a clear relationship between events that change our life situation and the onset of illness. These events can be anything from moving to a new home or getting married to being sued or being involved in a major traffic accident. Life events require adjustments in patterns of behavior and we often experience such adjustments as stressful.

As I've mentioned, perhaps the most significant life event is loss (actual, potential, or imagined) of a loved one. It can give rise to an emotional response of hopelessness and helplessness that results in our literally "giving up." When this happens, we can no longer cope, psychologically and biologically, with environmental demands. If we have a predisposition for a disease, then being in this psychological state makes the disease more likely to occur because our bodies are less capable of dealing effectively with the processes that give rise to the disease.

Studies have shown that life events often cluster to a statistically significant degree in the two-year period preceding illness, and that the onset of an illness can be predicted when a number of life events coincide. As we'll discuss in a moment, these results have led to attempts to quantify the impact of life changes and to identify the exact nature of the correlation with disease onset.

How Stress Causes Illness

There can be no doubt that there is a definite relationship between stress and illness. Although the exact nature of that relationship is not yet understood, a number of ideas have been suggested.

Early theories tried to connect different illnesses with specific types of emotional conflict or personality and body types. According to these theories, certain body types and temperaments would be more likely to develop one physical disease under stress than others. However, there is little agreement among the experts about what correlates with what.

Selye, in defining the general adaptation syndrome (GAS) that I mentioned earlier, has more to say on the subject. He maintains that the biological reactions accompanying the GAS result in both short- and long-term adverse physical changes. He calls these changes diseases of adaptation, since they are the outcome of a system of defenses against threatening stimuli.

The disease process is thought to arise as a result of factors such as: (a) The physiological effect of certain hormones from the adrenal and pituitary glands; (b) the impact of the inflammation process; and (c) a general state of lowered resistance. The actual disease that manifests itself depends on a range of factors, including genetics, physical weakness, and even specifically learned bodily responses.

The GAS helps explain the effects of life changes or events on health. Life changes require adjustments that could produce physiological reactions, and sustained and unsuccessful attempts at coping with life could lower bodily resistance and enhance the probability of illness. Thus, the more frequent and severe the life changes we experience, the more likely we are to become ill.

With these theories in mind, let's move on to discuss the ways that stress tends to manifest itself; then the rest of the book will deal with how to control stress and the diseases it causes.

THREE

How to Recognize Stress

S tress can affect our lives in many ways, and it is impossible to talk about them all here. However, when the level of stress goes beyond the point of being a healthy stimulant and starts to adversely affect our health, it usually takes the form of what doctors call "anxiety." Let's look at anxiety for a moment.

ANXIETY

Anxiety comprises various combinations of mental and physical symptoms that occur either in attacks (panic) or as a persisting state. It is often described in the following terms:

1. An emotional state colored with the experienced quality of fear.

2. An unpleasant emotion that may be accompanied by a feeling of impending doom.

3. A feeling directed toward the future, associated with a perceived threat of some kind.

4. An experience of bodily discomfort and actual bodily disturbance.

There may be no recognizable basis for the fear or feeling of threat, or the actual stimulus may be completely out of proportion to the emotion it provokes. Nevertheless, the symptoms it provokes are very real.

For some people, anxiety takes the form of recurrent attacks that, though they occur unpredictably, may become associated with specific situations. They start with a sudden, intense apprehension, often combined with a feeling of impending doom and sometimes with feelings of unreality. Any of the body symptoms described below may occur. An "anticipatory fear" of loss of control often develops, so that the person experiencing the attack becomes afraid of, for example, being left alone in public places. The anticipatory fear may itself precipitate other symptoms that escalate the attack.

Symptoms of Anxiety

There is not just one anxiety symptom. A whole range of reactions, listed in Table 1, has been associated with tension and anxiety.

Table 1: Symptoms of Anxiety

Anxious Mood:

Worrying	Anticipation of the worst
Apprehension (fearful anticipation)	Irritability

Fears of:

The dark	Strangers
Being left alone	Large animals
Traffic	Crowds

Intellectual (Cognitive) Symptoms:

Difficulty in concentration	Poor memory

Depressed Mood:

Loss of interest	Lack of pleasure in hobbies
Depression	Early waking
Diurnal swing	

General Body Sensations:

Tinnitus (noises in ear)	Blurred vision
Hot and cold flushes	Feelings of weakness
Prickling sensations	

Respiratory Symptoms:

Pressure or constriction in chest	Feelings of choking
Tightness of breath	Sighing

Genitourinary Symptoms:

Frequency of urination

Suppressed periods

Frigidity

Premature ejaculation

Impotence

Urgency of urination

Excessive bleeding during period

Loss of erection

Physiological Accompaniments of Behavior:

Tremor of hands

Strained face

Swallowing

Sweating

Furrowed brow

Facial pallor

Belching

Eyelid twitching

Tension:

Feelings of tension

Inability to relax

Easily moved to tears

Feelings of restlessness

Fatigue

Startled response

Trembling

Insomnia:

Difficulty in falling asleep

Unsatisfying sleep and fatigue on waking

Night terrors

Broken sleep

Dreams

Nightmares

General Somatic (Muscular) Symptoms:

Muscular aches and pains

Muscular twitching

Muscular stiffness

Grinding teeth

Heart Symptoms:

Tachycardia

Pain in chest

Feelings of faintness

Palpitations

Throbbing of vessels

Skipped heartbeats

Gastrointestinal Symptoms:

Difficulty in swallowing

Indigestion

Heartburn

Looseness of bowels

Constipation

Wind

Burps

Feelings of bloating

Loss of weight

Autonomic Symptoms:

Dry mouth

Pallor

Giddiness

Flushing

Tendency to sweat

Raising of hair

Adapted from: Hamilton, M. "The Assessment of Anxiety States by Rating," British Journal of Medical Psychology, 32, 1959, pp 50-55.

Anxiety-producing Life Events

Later in the book, a whole range of specific techniques will be discussed and herbal remedies suggested that will help with problems when they arise, but we needn't wait for the physical signs of stress to appear before we actively move toward ease in our lives. In the meantime, it is worth taking a closer look at some of the life events that predictably cause problems. To this end, a scale showing the relative anxiety-producing impact of certain life events is given in Table 2. The units on the scale are called "life change units" and give some indication of the chances of that particular event causing us problems. The higher the number of units, the higher the probability that we will experience stress and perhaps illness. Of course, a particular event will have more impact on some people than on others. Even so, the scale provides some valuable insights.

Table 2: The Relative Anxiety-producing Impact of Certain Life Events

Life Event	Impact in Life Change Units
1. Death of spouse	100
2. Divorce	73
3. Separation	65
4. Detention in jail	63
5. Death of close family member	63
6. Major personal injury or illness	53
7. Marriage	50
8. Loss of job	47
9. Marital reconciliation	45
10. Retirement	45
11. Major change in health or behavior of family member	44
12. Pregnancy	40
13. Sexual difficulties	39
14. New family member (through birth, adoption, relative moving in, etc.)	39
15. Major business readjustment	39
16. Major change in finances (lot better off or lot worse off)	38

17. Death of close friend	37
18. Change in line of work	36
19. Major change in number of arguments with spouse (lot more or lot less regarding children, personal habits, etc.)	35
20. New mortgage	31
21. Foreclosure on mortgage or loan	30
22. Major change in responsibilities at work	29
23. Child leaving home	29
24. In-law troubles	29
25. Outstanding personal achievement	28
26. Wife beginning or stopping work outside home	26
27. Beginning or end of formal schooling	26
28. Major change in living conditions (building new house, deterioration of home, etc.)	25
29. Change in personal habits (dress, etc.)	24
30. Troubles with boss	23
31. Major change in working hours or conditions	20
32. Change to new school	20
33. Change in usual type and/or amount of recreation	19
34. Major change in social activities	18
35. New loan	17
36. Major change in eating habits	15
37. Taking a vacation	13
38. Christmas	12

Adapted from: Holmes, T. and Rahne, "The Social Readjustment Rating Scale," Journal of Psychosomatic Research, 11, 1967, pp. 213-18.

This scale has been suggested as a tool for self-evaluation in the management of stress. Dr. Thomas Holmes has come up with these guidelines for its use:

1. Become familiar with the life events and the amount of change they may require. With practice, you can recognize life events when they happen.

2. Think about the meaning of the event for you and try to identify some of the feelings you experience.

3. Think about the different ways you might best adjust to the event.

4. Take your time in arriving at decisions.

5. If possible, anticipate life changes and plan for them well in advance.

6. Pace yourself, even if you are in a hurry.

7. Look at the accomplishment of a task as a part of daily living and avoid looking at each achievement as a "stopping point" or as a time for letting down.

8. Remember, the more changes that occur in your life, the more likely you are to get sick. Almost 80 percent of the people who experience more than 300 life change units in one year get sick, and with 150 to 299 life change units, about 50 percent get sick. However, with less than 150 life change units, only about 30 percent get sick. So the higher the score, the more you should take care of yourself!

The important point to bear in mind is that stress, tension, and anxiety are sometimes predictable. Don't be a victim! Recognize when you are moving into particularly difficult periods in your life and take steps to actively ease their impact. You can do this by using some of the herbal remedies discussed in the next chapter, but you should also take care of your body. Should you get some exercise or a massage? Is your diet providing enough B vitamins to help you cope with the extra stress? Preparing for the pressure will go a long way toward decreasing its impact on you.

FOUR

Controlling Stress:
An Overview

There is much that can be done to ease the impact of stress and lessen the weight of the anxiety and tension we so often carry around with us. However, the very range of approaches that we have to choose from can itself become a source of stress! Where should we turn for help? Which therapy should we use? These are always difficult questions, and they are even more difficult to answer when we are not feeling at our best.

The different therapies are only ways of helping us find the peace that is in us anyway. We are all in fact our own healers. The key is an inner attitude of taking responsibility for the quality of our own lives. We can seek aid from "experts," be they medical doctors, herbalists, or alternative-therapy practitioners, but the responsibility for healing can never be truly handed to another. Healing comes from within and is inherent to being alive. It is rarely an act of consciously harnessing inner energy, but it is always an expression of our inner power.

Healing can be facilitated by various tools and techniques. However, these techniques do not heal us; they can only aid in the healing process. Each of them embodies a profound truth and a great gift of healing wisdom, but humanity is very complex and our ills are a microcosm of that complexity. We need to build bridges between the therapies so that we can move toward a more holistic approach to health. In this chapter, I offer a simple model showing how we might integrate the various approaches to health and wholeness so that inner peace can become an active part of our lives.

The many healing techniques available to us, which often appear to contradict each other, can be seen as an ecological system of therapies. In this system, connections can be made between different branches of healing to produce a unique blend of therapies that is ideally suited to a particular person; a different blend would be right for someone else. The key to health and wholeness is finding the combination that will evoke the healing power of inner peace.

THE FOUR BRANCHES OF HEALING

Four branches of healing can be identified: medicine, body work, psychotherapy, and spiritual integration. Each of these branches consists of several specific therapies, many of which could be part of more than one of the four branches. I have tried to show the relationships between the branches in the model in Figure 1. As you can see, the model resembles a geodesic web of related therapies that we can call upon to facilitate the process of self-healing. While the whole model has limitations (for one thing, it's two-dimensional rather than multi-dimensional), it highlights a pattern of relationships, which is the vital point.

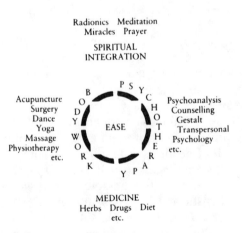

Figure 1. The relationships between the four branches of healing techniques

In the rest of this chapter, we'll take a brief look at each of the branches of therapy, starting with medicine. Specific therapies will be discussed in more detail in subsequent chapters.

Medicine

I use the term medicine to mean anything that is taken. In this context, medicine includes herbs, chemical drugs, homeopathic remedies, diet, Bach flower remedies, and aromatherapy. It may seem strange to group herbs and drugs together, but they are all part of the diversity and richness of our planet. Hydrocortisone, meadowsweet, and Bach flower remedies are all produced from the body of the earth in one way or another. There is nothing universally bad about drugs or universally good about herbs. Let us be thankful for the choice. The use of drugs to stop a biochemical disease process is at times valid and life-saving, but to be human is to be much more than a combination of biological functions and the removal of symptoms is not the same as being healed.

Body Work

Body-work theories recognize that the physical body has a deep wisdom of its own that goes beyond the mind's comprehension. A vast range of healing techniques focus on the body, with surgery being perhaps the most mechanical and invasive. I do not mean to deny surgery's undoubted power in saving and enhancing life, but I do want to point out the limitations inherent in a technique that is purely a response to already established pathology. Fortunately, we have many other, less rigorous body-work approaches available to us. I don't want to debate the pros and cons of each therapy here; instead, my goal is to begin painting a broad picture of the relationships between them. For example, acupuncture offers a profound way of balancing body energies and, as the Chinese have shown us, it has a lot to offer in combination with herbal treatment. Other very different approaches to the body include the manipulative methods, such as osteopathy, chiropractic, and physiotherapy; and in the context of stress management, body-work tools such as yoga, the Alexander technique, Feldenkrais, exercise, and dance take on a primary role. Massage, with its many variations, also has a wonderful contribution to make.

Psychotherapy

Psychotherapy and counseling are increasingly relevant in our stressed and insane times, and in our society the work of counselors is greatly undervalued. Much pain and trauma is the result of emotional and mental problems, which we can fortunately tackle with techniques developed to enhance inner knowledge and psychological integration. These techniques include the traditional but limited approach of psychoanalysis, as well as the more holistic techniques of humanistic and transpersonal psychology, such as gestalt and psychosynthesis. The human-potential movement, with its great proliferation of techniques, also has much to offer in a broad approach to healing.

Spiritual Integration

Inherent in a holistic view of humanity is the perception of an integrating center, a spiritual core, a source of life and love. To the spiritually orientated, disease might be viewed as the result of an inhibited soul life. For the purposes of healing, there are ways in which we can be open to our spiritual selves and ways in which others can affect our "spiritual bodies," including through prayer, meditation, spiritual healing, and radionics. It is here that I would include the mystery of "miracles," the undoubtedly miraculous healing of incurable conditions. The implications of such miracles go way beyond the focus of this book, but let us thank God that they are real!

THE RIGHT COMBINATION

The network of therapies described by my model provides a spectrum of insights that recognizes that we are all unique individuals. Each of us will find one approach or group of approaches more beneficial than others. For some of us, a combination of herbal medicine, osteopathy, and psychotherapy may be the most helpful in our attempts to be healthy and whole, while for others, surgery and drugs may be needed. All combinations are valid as we search for the key that will release our powers of self-healing and inner peace.

This small model, which attempts to show the relationships between therapies, is but a part of a greater vision that is holistic healing. It is one example of a transformation that is taking place in Western ways of thinking. We live in times of change and chaos out of which a whole new paradigm, or pattern, of world view is slowly emerging.

What is Holistic Medicine?

As people in all fields of life explore the implications of a holistic and ecological world view, medicine and the healing arts are at the forefront. But what is holistic medicine, other than a "buzz word"?

Holistic medicine addresses the physical, mental, and spiritual aspects of those who come for care, viewing health as a positive state, not as the absence of disease. It emphasizes the uniqueness of the individual and the importance of tailoring treatment to meet each person's needs. The promotion of health and the prevention of disease are priorities, and the responsibility of each individual for his or her own health is stressed. In keeping with this philosophy, holistic medicine uses therapeutic approaches that mobilize the person's innate capacity for self-healing. While recognizing the occasional necessity for swift medical or surgical intervention, its emphasis is on understanding and self-help, on education and self-care, rather than on treatment and dependence.

A holistic approach to health care includes understanding and treating people in the context of their culture and community. A comprehension of those social and economic conditions that perpetuate ill health, and a commitment to changing them, are as much a part of holistic medicine as its emphasis on individual responsibility. Holistic medicine thus transforms its practitioners as well as its patients.

Herbal medicine has much to contribute to the development of holistic health care. As I've said, the use of herbs for healing brings us immediately in touch with our world in a profoundly deep and uplifting way. Thus, herbal medicine, while being a valid and effective healing tool, can also be part of a personal, and even social, transformation.

Such holistic perspectives suggest exciting ways in which health care can evolve, but for this to happen, the relationship between the complementary therapies and orthodox medicine must be developed. This will create a framework for fulfilling the expectations of health and well being that have been raised.

To help you select the right combination of therapies for the management of the stress, anxiety, and tension that are the basis for many modern diseases, we shall consider in the next chapters what some specific therapies have to offer, and how you can go about using them in practice. The main approach we shall consider is herbalism, but we will also briefly cover relaxation techniques, meditation, yoga, autogenic training, biofeedback, diet, dance, massage, and several other therapies. They will all be considered in the context of the four branches of healing described in this chapter, and in the context of a holistic approach to health and well being.

FIVE

Controlling Stress with Herbs and Related Remedies

W e will start our review of the ways to control stress by examining things that can be *taken*. *Herbal* remedies will be looked at in depth. Other related therapies touched on in this chapter will be Bach flower remedies, aromatherapy, homeopathy, and nutrition. However, stress must be approached on a broad front, so bear in mind that the information in this chapter complements that given about body work, psychological techniques, and spiritual integration in the following chapters.

HERBS

Herbs have been used as medicines for as long as humanity has been keeping written records. Every culture at every point in time has based its healing arts on plants. It is only very recently that Western approaches to medicine have moved to the one-sided, scientific view of illness that has promoted the development of chemical medicine. We have now become accustomed to "health" coming from a bottle of pills, and the idea that a wayside plant can help in times of trauma sounds too simple to be true. In the context of chemical medicine, herbal remedies are seen as sources of valuable "active ingredients;" the dandelion and the violet are "raw materials" – bags of chemicals. But herbs are much more than that. Plant remedies are nature's gift to a suffering humanity – an expression of our belonging in the world. In these times of alienation from each other and from nature,

they are an almost revolutionary reminder of humanity's one-
ness with nature.

There are several theories about how herbs work. For many
people, it is enough that they do! It is possible, however, to use
the insights of science to describe the pattern of relationships
involved. To do this, we must dip into the realms of geology,
evolutionary biology, and ecology.

The Gaia Hypothesis and Herbal Remedies

New insights into the workings of our planet as a whole give
us exciting opportunities to view ourselves from new perspectives. The work of the geochemist Jim Lovelock has shown us
that the earth is not a passive geophysical object but an active
participant in the creation of its own story – a living entity that
he named Gaia after the Greek goddess of the earth. Lovelock
has described Gaia as:

"... a complex entity involving the earth's biosphere, atmosphere, oceans, and soil; the totality constituting a feedback
system that seeks an optimal chemical and physical environment
on this planet. The maintenance of relatively constant conditions
occurs through active control." – Lovelock, J.E. *Gaia, A New Look
at Life on Earth*, Oxford University Press (1979)

This implies that our world is working actively as a whole to
create and maintain optimum conditions for life to thrive and
evolve. Human consciousness is an integral part of this evolutionary drive, and the opportunity lies before us to embrace our
role within the greater being of Gaia, our world. This idea is not
new; it has inspired the mystics of all ages. But we have finally
reached a point where this idea has become the stuff of science.

The scientific discipline known as ecology is showing us how
all that lives upon our planet is integrated and mutually dependent in a profound and complex way. With the concept of Gaia
in mind, evolution becomes as much an exercise in cooperation
as competition, both processes having contributed to the creation of the complex tapestry of today's ecology. The ecosystem
can only be understood as a whole. It is a self-sustaining system, supplying all that is needed by any part of the whole. In
fact, the needs of the parts have to be supplied by the system

because there is nothing outside it. If the system does not take care of itself, it cannot survive. Humanity has survived and flourished without drug therapy and without the wonders of high-tech surgery. Moreover, we have produced empires, great art, and the very science that has given us modern medicine.

Herbs contain complex chemicals that are called secondary plant products because they play no apparent role in the life of the plant. Until recently, biochemists assumed that these chemicals were elaborate waste-disposal systems, but this hypothesis seems totally out of keeping with the genius of plants for efficiency and design. These chemicals are, in fact, the very ones that have such a marked action on human physiology.

This is not merely a fortuitous accident, but the hallmark of Gaia – evidence of a planetary circulation of energy, life, and healing. By eating plants or drinking herb teas, we link ourselves to a circulatory system within the biosphere and to the energy source of the sun. The secondary plant products take part in this planetary circulation, helping humanity and thus the health of the whole planet. Through plants – as food or as medicine – we get in touch with the vitality of our world.

Active Ingredients or Whole Plants?

The valuable and potent chemicals in plants are what pharmacists consider to be their active ingredients, and vast amounts of money go into the search for potential new ways to use these chemicals to produce drugs. But the isolation and synthesis of specific active ingredients, such as aspirin from willow bark and digoxin from foxglove, is a mistake and may even be harmful. In the plants themselves, these powerful constituents are balanced and made accessible to the body by the numerous other constituents present.

For example, the Chinese herb ma huang (Ephedra sinica) contains an alkaloid called ephedrine, which, in addition to alleviating conditions such as asthma, raises blood pressure if given as an extracted drug. However, the plant also contains six other alkaloids, one of which actually prevents a rise in blood pressure and an increase in heart rate. The isolated drug is dangerous, but the whole plant is balanced by nature to make a safer remedy. Why, then, don't the chemists extract all seven alkaloids? They clearly don't trust nature's own skills in balancing herbal remedies! Another example is the dandelion leaf, a potent and useful diuretic that requires none of the potassium supplements usually essential with conventional drug diuretics, which have potassium loss as their side effect. The leaves are so rich in this essential mineral that dandelion leaves are a perfectly balanced remedy, leaving the body with a healthy net increase in potassium.

This reveals the core of the benefit of herbal remedies when treating stress and anxiety. Not only do these remedies contain "active ingredients" to calm the nerves or lift depression, but they also gently aid the whole body to be at ease and regain health.

Can we be reduced to the level of molecules and can our anxieties be interpreted as purely biochemical phenomena? Of course not. The use of potent drugs to suppress and block the expression of tension does nothing to remedy the underlying causes of the problem. The human body surpasses description in the beauty and dynamic complexity of its form and function, in its potential and creativity. On the level of physical form, the body is indeed biochemical, but its organization transcends the realms of chemical medicine. Even if we could comprehend its molecular complexities, we would not be any nearer to knowing what makes us human. The powerful, integrating force at work within us – call it life, vital force, or the spark of life – is involved with us on all levels, not just the biochemical. Herbal medicine recognizes this life force and uses the planet's gift of herbs to augment this force, bringing about a deep healing and not simply the relief of symptoms.

The Nervous System and Herbal Remedies

In no other system of the body is the connection between the physical and psychological aspects of our being as apparent as in the nervous system. Clearly, the tissue of the nervous system is part of the physical makeup of the body but, just as clearly, all psychological processes also take place in the nervous system. Therefore, if there is "dis-ease" on the psychological level, it will be reflected on the physiological level.

As I've said, orthodox medicine tends to reduce psychological problems to the mere biochemical level, and assumes that "appropriate" drugs will sort out or at least hide the problem sufficiently to allow "normal" life to continue. Interestingly enough, some techniques in the field of complementary medicine assume or imply the other extreme: namely, that psychological factors are the cause of all disease. Treatment of the psyche is, therefore, the only appropriate way of healing, and will take care of any physical problem. By bringing these two reductionist views together, we come closer to a holistic approach. A holistic approach to healing acknowledges the interconnectedness of physiological and psychological factors, and regards the nervous system and its functions as a vital element in the treatment of the whole being. To be truly healthy, we have to take care of our physical health through the right diet and life style, but we are also responsible for taking care of our emotional, mental, and spiritual life. We should endeavor to live in a fulfilling, nurturing environment that supports emotional stability. Our thoughts should be creative and life-enhancing, open to the free flow of intuition and imagination, rather than conceptually rigid. And we should stay open to the free flow of the higher energies of our souls, without which health is impossible.

Herbal medicine can be an ecologically and spiritually integrative tool that is an ideal counterpart on the physical level for therapeutic techniques on the psychological level. Herbs can benefit the nervous system in a number of ways, in addition to the rather simplistic ones of stimulation and relaxation. In Western herbalism today, it is common to differentiate between three kinds of herbs that act on the nervous system, collectively called nervines. These are nervine tonics, nervine relaxants, and nervine stimulants. We'll look at each of these in turn. Bear in mind that the herbal remedies mentioned here in a broad context are also discussed in greater depth in the last chapter of the book.

Nervine tonics

Perhaps the most important contribution herbal medicine can make in the whole area of stress and anxiety management is in strengthening and "feeding" the nervous system. In cases of shock, stress, or nervous debility, the nervine tonics can be used to strengthen and restore the tissues; there is no need to resort to tranquillizers or other drugs to ease anxiety or depression. In many other "nerve" problems, the nervine tonics can also be invaluable.

Surprising as it may seem, one of the best and certainly one of the most widely applicable remedies for feeding nervous tissue is common oats, which can either be taken in the form of tinctures, combined as needed with relaxants, stimulants or any other indicated remedy, or can simply be eaten as cooked oatmeal. The oats must be old-fashioned whole oat groats; instant or rolled oatflakes do not have the plant's original integrity, and are useless here.

Two other remedies also have a profound action upon the body as a whole. These are ginseng and Siberian ginseng. The term "adaptogen" has been coined to describe their undoubted ability to help the whole body and the mind cope with the demands made upon them.

Other nervine tonics that have a relaxing as well as a strengthening effect include damiana, scullcap, vervain, and wood betony. Of these, scullcap is often the most effective, particularly for problems related to stress.

Nervine relaxants

In cases of stress and tension, the nervine relaxants can help a lot. They are the closest natural alternative to orthodox medicine's tranquillizers, but should always be used in a broad holistic way. Too much tranquillizing, even if achieved through a herbal remedy, can in time deplete the whole nervous system.

The following list is far from complete but includes the main restoratives of the nervine-relaxant category:

Black cohosh	Lemon balm
Black haw	Lime blossom
California poppy	Mistletoe
Chamomile	Motherwort
Cramp bark	Pasque flower
Hops	Passionflower
Hyssop	Rosemary
Jamaica dogwood	St. John's wort
Lady's slipper	Scullcap
Lavender	Valerian

Many of the relaxants on this list also have other properties and can be selected to aid in related problems. This is one of the great benefits of using herbal remedies to help with stress and anxiety problems, since the physical symptoms that so often accompany anxiety may well be treated with the same herbs chosen to treat the anxiety.

The herbs mentioned so far work directly on the nervous system. The antispasmodic herbs, which affect the peripheral nerves and the muscle tissue, can also be used for their indirect relaxing effect on the system, since when the physical body is at ease, psychological ease is promoted. Different antispasmodic herbs relax and ease different tissues of the body. It is worth studying the herbal at the end of this book to see which herbs have this property in addition to their main one.

Many of the nervine relaxants also have an antispasmodic action. By far the most important and safe are cramp bark, valerian, and wild haw.

Demulcent plants can also be used in conjunction with nervine relaxants, as they soothe irritated tissue and promote healing.

Nervine stimulants

Direct stimulation of the nervous tissue is not very often needed in our hyperactive times. It is usually more appropriate to stimulate the body's innate vitality with the help of nervine or even digestive tonics, which work by augmenting bodily harmony and thus have a much deeper and longer-lasting effect than nervine stimulants. Herbalists placed much more emphasis on stimulant herbs in the last century than they do now – perhaps a sign that today's world is supplying us with more than enough stimulus.

When direct nervine stimulation is indicated, the best herb to use is kola, though coffee, mate, and black tea may also be used. A problem with these common stimulants is that they have a number of side effects and can themselves cause minor psychological upsets that can lead to anxiety and tension. Although short-term use is appropriate at times, daily cups of strong coffee can cause too many problems to list here.

Some of the herbs that are rich in volatile oils are also valuable stimulants, one of the most common and best being peppermint.

The bitter herbs can have a positive effect on the nervous system through their general stimulation of the metabolism. Such herbs as wormwood and mugwort come to mind.

Herbal Allies

From this apparently large and confusing list of effective remedies, we each need to select the ones appropriate for ourselves. Each of us will find that particular herbs suit us better than others. Such herbs have been called "herbal allies." There is no way for me to give instructions about how to find your allies, but once found, they will act in a deep and profound way that is especially helpful in easing the impact of stress and general anxiety, as well as any specific health problems you may have.

Herbal Remedies for Daily Use

If you know that a period of stress and strain is about to fill your life with its usual basket of goodies, it is worth preparing for it ahead of time. Certain herbs, diet, and life-style changes will minimize the impact. We've already discussed life events and the fact that it is possible to prepare for them; here, we shall discuss preparing for stress with herbal aids.

A number of herbs can be used regularly as gentle relaxants. They can be drunk as teas or cold drinks, infused in massage oil, and used in relaxing foot baths or even full baths. Some can be used to make quite delicious wines, but this could be an herbal way to become an alcoholic, so use this method with discretion! Different ways of preparing the herbs are described in more detail in Chapter 9, "How to Prepare Herbal Remedies."

Some of the plants that can be used as safe, daily easers of stress and calmers of anxiety are listed below. Taste and general intuition may tell you which is the most suitable to use. The herbal chapter at the end of the book contains much more detailed information.

BALM: A very traditional English herb that graced Elizabethan gardens and can be grown in city window boxes. Not only visually aesthetic but has an aroma that is strongly reminiscent of lemons and geraniums. This aroma is imparted into tea made with balm and is partially responsible for its action. In addition to its relaxing action, it settles the stomach and calms most mild digestive upsets.

CHAMOMILE: A popular relaxing herb that also has many beneficial effects on the digestive system. An "acquired taste."

LAVENDER: A wonderful herb in all ways. The very fact that nature has provided us with this plant should give us the message that underneath all our problems, life is very good indeed!

LIME BLOSSOM: A valuable and pleasant tea for easing and relaxing the stresses of the day. Acts on the circulatory system and is good for people with high blood pressure.

OATS: It may seem surprising that this food should be included in a list of herbs, but oats should be part of the diet of anyone under stress.

SCULLCAP: A strong relaxing remedy that can be used if deeper relaxation is needed.

VALERIAN: Even stronger than scullcap and discussed in more detail later.

WOOD BETONY: A common wild herb that eases away daily tensions, especially those that cause headaches.

In addition to taking herbal remedies, it is important to ensure that your food is feeding your body, and especially your nervous system, well. Guidelines for good diet are given later. For now I'll just mention that a vitamin supplement may be required in times of stress. A daily supplement of the B-complex vitamins, perhaps combined with vitamin C, would be most beneficial.

As well as responding to stress in a healthy way – enjoying herbs and improving your diet – try to reduce the stress itself. This is sometimes impossible, but don't put up with something or someone just because they are there. You can change and you can change your life. It helps to re-evaluate your choices. Are you doing what you really want to do? If not, what would you rather be doing? Give yourself permission to ask some searching questions about yourself and your life-style. Don't censor any of the answers that may come up! After pinpointing your inner motivations you can choose what you do about them. If changing is too difficult or painful, you are free to not change. Instead, you may choose to use herbs and, perhaps, counseling to help ease the strain so you can live a less tense and anxious life. However, if you choose to change, herbal medicine if used wisely can aid you in the process of transformation.

Herbal Remedies for Chronic Stress

The line between chronic stress and the daily levels we all seem to put up with is fuzzy. A gentle soul with not too strong a constitution will cross the line sooner than a stronger person who copes well. Neither of these extremes of personality is "better" than the other; they merely reflect the fact that we live in a world of human diversity. That's sometimes a joy and sometimes an actual cause of stress!

The advice given for daily stress relief holds for chronic stress, but in addition the following two remedies should become staples:

GINSENG: A dried root that is renowned for its ability to improve the balance of bodily functions and for its ability to variously stimulate and relax the nervous system.

SIBERIAN GINSENG: Also a dried root that is even more stimulating in action than ginseng. Aids and supports the whole of the hormonal system, which deals with the impact of stress.

There is no close botanical relationship between these two herbs; the similarity in names comes from commercial interests. They should not be taken together; choose one or the other, depending upon which suits you best.

Herbal Remedies for Immediate Relief

There are times in most people's lives when things get to be too much and the pain of existence builds to a crescendo. Immediate herbal relief may be needed in a whole range of traumatic situations – from being involved in a car accident to some personal emotional crisis. In all cases, herbs will take the edge off the trauma but will rarely remove it. At such times herbs can be only an aid – one element of the approach taken to deal with the difficulties being faced. This approach may also include seeking help from the various caring professions, going on vacation or on a retreat, or even checking into a hospital.

The plants that are capable of easing intense stress are considered dangerous in our society and because they are restricted drugs, they will not be discussed here. However, in addition to the herbs previously mentioned, the following remedies should be considered:

JAMAICA DOGWOOD: A pain reliever that reduces anxiety and facilitates relaxation and sleep.

LADY'S SLIPPER: Also called American valerian because it has similar properties.

PASSIONFLOWER: A good and safe remedy that will help with sleeplessness. Does not increase passion!

VALERIAN: A widely applicable and quite strong relaxing plant. In some sensitive people, has been known to cause agitation, but if it suits you, you can use it as strongly as you like. A sleep inducer at high dosage. Will also ease pain and help with digestive gas problems.

WILD LETTUCE: This plant is not to be confused with common lettuce! The strength of this mild tranquillizer unfortunately varies from plant to plant.

ANTISPASMODIC DROPS: A combination of several herbs, not all of which are nervines. Eases shock and trauma. A number of brands are available and it is easier to buy a bottle from a reputable herb supplier than to try and concoct them yourself. Take as directed on the label.

RESCUE REMEDY: One of the best treatments for shock available. Discussed in more detail in the section on Bach flower remedies.

Let us now move on to consider other remedies for stress that involve "things" that can be taken.

AROMATHERAPY

The fragrance of flowers is one of their most wonderful gifts to humanity, and in recent years the healing value of different aromas has been increasingly acknowledged. Plant oils are the basis of the aromas and are called essential oils. Chemically each plant has an amazing array of different specific oils that combine to produce the unique quality of each type of plant. Research has shown that the oils have a distinct effect upon the mind, as well as antiseptic and other properties.

Aromatherapy, the use of essential oils, is a vast field and anyone interested in studying further will find recommended books in the bibliography. Here, we will just briefly consider the oils that may help in easing stress and the ways in which they may be used. Because the oils are usually massaged into the skin, this therapy could have been included in the body-work section of the next chapter. However, the oils are absorbed by the skin and their effect is internal, so we will look at them in this chapter instead.

The oils may be used for the whole spectrum of human ills, including the physical and mental problems that can result from stress. Many oils have strong antiseptic and antibacterial properties. The application of chamomile and lavender oils to infected wounds can be as effective as the use of phenol. Spraying eucalyptus oil will purify the air and therefore has a role to play in any sickroom. Examples of essential oils that can be used for psychological problems are orange flower for anxiety, worry, or insomnia; rose for stress and depression (it is also reputed to ease hangovers!); and basil, rosemary, and patchouli for stimulating mental clarity, concentration, and memory.

Essential oils are most effective if used as part of a whole program for restoring health and ease. The oils should never be ingested except under the guidance of a skilled medical herbalist or aromatherapist.

Each of the oils listed below has a vast range of actions; however, here I will just mention their use for stress-related problems. Only a small selection is given; nature is truly abundant in her gifts and there is not room to acknowledge them all.

BASIL: A refreshing and stimulating oil. Basil is a nerve tonic that aids concentration and clarifies the mind.

CHAMOMILE: Soothing and calming for anxiety. Will relax muscles as well as act as an anti-inflammatory agent. For insomnia use in a late bath.

CLARY SAGE: A good relaxing oil with euphoric effects on sensitive people! May help with insomnia.

HYSSOP: A mild sedative and general nerve tonic that helps regulate blood pressure, whether high or low.

JASMINE: A wonderful aroma that is antidepressant and supposedly a sensual stimulant. Eases pain in the whole of the female reproductive system.

LAVENDER: If you could have only one oil, let it be lavender! It relaxes and eases aches and pains. It has a whole range of positive physical actions, but is especially useful for migraines and headaches.

MARJORAM: Useful for anxiety, grief, and insomnia as well as easing muscular, menstrual, and rheumatic pains. May help with migraine. A very warming remedy.

ORANGE FLOWER ABSOLUTE: A beautiful strong aroma that is quite effective for anxiety and its associated symptoms, such as palpitations. Will ease depression as well. Good for shock and fear.

PATCHOULI: A stimulant to the nerves that lifts anxiety and depression. Has a reputation as an aphrodisiac.

PINE: Primarily an antiseptic oil, but helps clear the mind. Also of benefit in mental fatigue.

ROSE: Very soothing for the nerves. An antidepressant. Can calm anger and alleviate hangovers.

ROSEMARY: An invigorating oil that may stimulate a weak memory and general dullness. Helpful for headaches.

SANDALWOOD: A calming and refreshing oil that eases anxiety and nervous tension.

VERBENA: An excellent nerve tonic that eases and strengthens at the same time. For all anxiety problems, especially palpitations and dizziness. An insect repellent.

YLANG-YLANG: A sweet, exotic scent that is supposedly aphrodisiac. Stimulates the senses and brings about a sense of well being. Good for anxiety, tension, and anger.

How To Use Essential Oils

As already pointed out, while they should not be ingested, there is a whole range of ways to benefit from these wonderful oils. The following are the best methods to help with stress problems. There are other ways of using the oils for getting rid of infections and easing muscular pains.

Massage oils

The aromatic oils blend well with any bland massage oil, giving you the opportunity to experiment and learn what is most appropriate for you. Examples of possible mixtures are 10 to 12 drops of essential oil to 20 ml of almond oil, or 60 drops to 100 ml of almond oil.

Bath oils

Add 5 to 10 drops of oil to a full bath. This way, you absorb the aroma not only through the skin but also by inhaling.

Perfumes

Any of the pleasant fragrances may be used as perfumes, alone or blended.

Vaporization

A few drops can be added to a heat source, such as a radiator or small bowl of hot water. All the oils evaporate easily.

Cologne

Add 3 drops of essential oil to 100 ml of distilled water. Keep the mixture in a dark, airtight bottle. It will stay fresh for a few weeks.

BACH FLOWER THERAPY

The Bach flower remedies represent an approach to herbalism that is an alchemical amalgam of the spiritual essence of the flower in cooperation with the emotional/mental need of the person. They are not used directly for physical illness, but for the person's worry, apprehension, hopelessness, fear, irritability, and so on. As we have seen, a person's psychic state has a major bearing on the causation, development, and cure of any physical illness. The remedies appear to work with the lifeforce, allowing it to flow freely through or around any block that illness puts in its way and so speeding healing and a return to wholeness. Just as aromatherapy could have been included in the body-work section in Chapter 6, so the Bach remedies could have been included in that chapter's integration section.

The remedies were developed by Dr. Edward Bach, who lived from 1880 to 1936. The story of how he developed them is wonderful indeed and worth reading about. (The contact address for further information about the remedies is: Ellon (Bach USA), 463 Rockaway Ave, Valley Stream, NY 11580.) Bach divided the negative states of mind from which we so often suffer into seven major categories: apprehension, indecision, loneliness, insufficient interest in circumstances, oversensitivity, despondency and despair, and excessive concern for others. To help us deal with these states, he found 38 flowers that are ideal for self-use, are inherently benign in action, have no unpleasant reactions, and can be used by anyone. The dose is simply a few drops of the special flower extracts in water.

I have adapted the following list from a brief guide produced by the Bach Centre in England to give you an idea of the uses of the different flower remedies:

AGRIMONY: For those who suffer inner torture which they try to hide behind a facade of cheerfulness.

ASPEN: For apprehension, foreboding, and fears of unknown origin.

BEECH: For those who are arrogant, critical, and intolerant of others.

CENTAURY: For weakness of will in those who let themselves be imposed upon, who become subservient, and who have difficulty saying "no."

CERATO: For those who doubt their own judgment and overly seek the advice of others. For those who are often influenced and misguided.

CHERRY PLUM: For a fear of mental collapse, desperation, or loss of control. For vicious rages.

CHESTNUT BUD: For those who refuse to learn by experience and continually repeat the same mistakes.

CHICORY: For the overpossessive and those who demand attention. For selfishness. For those who like others to conform to their standards and those who often make martyrs of themselves.

CLEMATIS: For the indifferent, inattentive, dreamy, and absent-minded. For those who mentally escape from reality.

CRAB APPLE: A cleanser for those who feel unclean or ashamed of their ailments. For self-disgust and the house-proud.

ELM: For those who are temporarily overcome by responsibility or inadequacy, though they are normally very capable.

GENTIAN: For the despondent, easily discouraged, and dejected.

GORSE: For extreme hopelessness.

HEATHER: For those who are obsessed with their own troubles and experiences. For poor listeners.

HOLLY: For those who are jealous, envious, revengeful, and suspicious. For those who hate.

HONEYSUCKLE: For those with nostalgia who constantly dwell in the past. Also for homesickness.

HORNBEAM: For procrastination and the "Monday morning" feeling.

IMPATIENS: For impatience and irritability.

LARCH: For despondency due to lack of self-confidence. For those who expect failure, so fail to make an attempt. For those who feel inferior though they have the ability.

MIMULUS: For fear of known things, shyness, and timidity.

MUSTARD: For deep gloom that descends for no known reason but that can lift just as suddenly. For melancholy.

OAK: For determination. For those who struggle on in illness and against adversity, despite setbacks. For plodders.

OLIVE: For exhaustion. For those who are drained of energy and for whom everything is an effort.

PINE: For feelings of guilt. For those who blame themselves for the mistakes of others and feel unworthy.

RED CHESTNUT: For excessive fear and concern for people dear to us.

ROCK ROSE: For terror, extreme fear, or panic.

ROCK WATER: For those who are hard on themselves, rigid-minded, and self-denying.

SCLERANTHUS: For uncertainty, indecision, and vacillation.

STAR OF BETHLEHEM: For the effects of bad news or fright following an accident.

SWEET CHESTNUT: For the anguish of those who have reached the limits of endurance and absolute dejection.

VERVAIN: For overenthusiasm, overeffort, and straining. For the fanatical.

VINE: For those who are dominating, inflexible, ambitious, and autocratic. For arrogance and pride.

WALNUT: For protection from powerful influences. Helps adjustment to any transition or change, such as menopause or divorce.

WATER VIOLET: For the proud, reserved, and "superior."

WHITE CHESTNUT: For persistent unwanted thoughts, preoccupation with a worry or event, and mental arguments.

WILD OAT: Helps determine one's intended path in life.

WILD ROSE: For resignation and apathy. For drifters who accept their lot, making little effort for improvement.

WILLOW: For resentment and bitterness. For those with a "poor me" attitude.

Rescue Remedy

Rescue remedy is a combination of cherry plum, clematis, impatiens, rock rose, and star of Bethlehem. It is an all-purpose, emergency composite that can be used to treat the effects on a sufferer of serious news, bereavement, terror, severe mental trauma, a feeling of desperation, a numbed, bemused state of mind, or any other stress. It is taken orally, at a dose of about four drops in a glass of water.

HOMEOPATHY

Homeopathy is one of the more established complementary therapies but perhaps one of the least understood. As a broad medical approach it has much to offer, both in treating illness and helping prevent disease. It would appear that a skilled homeopathic practitioner can treat an individual at a deep constitutional level, thereby promoting health and wholeness on all levels.

It is impossible to talk here about the homeopathic remedies for stress and anxiety. Many specific remedies might help, but they all depend upon a broader picture of physical health, general medical history, personality type, and so on. To use the homeopathic remedies correctly and effectively involves comprehending what is known as the "symptoms picture." It takes years of study and experience for a skilled homeopathic practitioner to gain facility and ease with matching different remedies to different people.

Homeopathic treatment is of undoubted value and benefit, but a critical ingredient is the skill, training, and perception of the practitioner. Therefore, no remedies will be recommended here. Self-treatment with homeopathic pills is to be avoided.

DIET

By now everyone has heard the expression "You are what you eat." Nowhere is this more true than in a person who is under stress and suffering subsequent tension. Ideally, the food we eat and the way we eat it supplies us with all the nutrition we need and with a time of relaxation in which to digest it. Most people are not ideal, however! The usual diet of our society has been deplored by everyone from dieticians to the government, so rather than add my own comments, I will focus on how to ensure that the nervous system, as well as the whole body and the mind, is adequately fed.

One point: avoid fad diets. They may be good for weight loss, but they are very bad for awareness and consciousness.

What to Eat

In general, a healthy diet is one that is rich in fresh, raw vegetables and fruits, with a small amount of good meat if you can morally justify it to yourself. A major problem with meat in stress-related conditions is the feed that has been given to the animals and the chemicals that may have been used to stimulate their growth. Much of current animal husbandry is straight out of a chemistry lab, something that we as consumers know little about.

The diet should also contain a fair proportion of roughage, but not buckets of bran! Wholegrain bread and a proportion of raw vegetables should provide the roughage you need.

A key to any dietary approach to health has to be the avoidance of artificial additives in any form – extremely difficult but vital. Additives include flavors, colors, and preservatives.

A good supply of the B-complex vitamins and vitamin C is essential. The C is available in fruits and most green vegetables, while the B is found in whole grains, eggs, some fish, molasses, and brewer's yeast.

Many foods should be avoided to help reduce anxiety and tension in general. As a priority, don't take any food or drink containing caffeine, which increases agitation; this means no coffee, tea, or chocolate. Too much red meat can also act as a physical stimulant and should probably be avoided. Alcohol has a deleterious effect on the nervous system, among other problems, and should be avoided, along with tobacco.

How to Eat

The way we eat affects our digestion of food. Eating should be a time of ease and peace. Here are some suggestions:

1. Eat small meals at regular intervals – every two or three hours if possible.
2. Eat your meals slowly and chew your food carefully.
3. Avoid rush and hurry before and after meals. Try to arrange a short rest before and after eating.

4. Sufficient sleep at night is important; aim for eight hours.

5. Remember that anxiety and worry can upset digestion.

6. Avoid large and heavy meals, fried foods and anything that disagrees with you.

7. Never smoke or drink before meals.

8. Drink only sparingly during meals but take plenty of fluids between meals.

Having looked briefly at controlling stress with herbs and related remedies, let's now move on to survey the other three branches of stress therapy.

SIX

Body Work

I n Chapter 4, I presented a model of the relationships between four branches of stress therapy. We've already looked at herbal and related remedies; in the following three chapters, I'll briefly cover the other three branches: body work, psychotherapy, and spiritual integration. Detailed discussion of these branches is beyond the scope of this book; indeed, each warrants a whole book in its own right! The goal of these chapters is to give you a "feel" for each of these branches of healing and a sense of how therapies can complement each other in the treatment of stress in general and of stress-induced diseases in particular.

The body takes the brunt of much of the stress that we carry around with us. Whole areas of psychology focus on body/mind interactions, and we now know that it is a mistake to even think of the body and the mind as separate entities. We have seen how psychosomatic illnesses are the grounding of psychological anxieties in physical forms. Turning body/mind interactions to our advantage, it is also possible to relax the mind by easing the tension stored in the muscles of the body. Many ways have been developed to do this, but we will discuss only a few. Relaxation techniques will be looked at in depth, followed by yoga, dance, the Alexander technique, and touch-based therapies such as massage. Finally, we'll talk about exercise in general.

RELAXATION

Perhaps the most important and yet the simplest tool we have available for reducing the impact of stress is relaxation exercises. When we are tense and on edge, and have been so for a while, the worst thing anyone can say to us is, "Relax; take it easy." That advice is guaranteed to put us even further on edge as we work at trying to relax! The sad fact is that few of us retain the innate skill of relaxation – a pity, but there it is. Relaxation is a skill that we must learn and practice.

There are vast ranges of relaxation techniques, some based on breathing, some on muscle control, some on visualization, and some that simply involve listening to music. It's a matter of finding which is most suitable for you. Of the many varieties of relaxation exercises that we could explore in this section, we will focus on three: muscle awareness, rhythmic breathing, and muscle contraction. The first, muscle awareness, is examined more closely than the others, to show the general approach you should take to doing this sort of exercise. Additional relaxation exercises are described later in this chapter in the section on psychotherapy techniques.

MUSCLE AWARENESS

The muscle-awareness technique was designed by Dr. Harold Geld simply to develop awareness of the larger muscles. It works most effectively if you let yourself be physically passive, yet mentally aware and alert. It is the act of conscious attention that allows the muscles to relax.

Initially, it is best to consciously practice this awareness at specific times, but gradually it will become automatic, unconscious, and continuous. Sometimes this muscle awareness is really all that's necessary for the brain's muscle-control centers to learn deep relaxation, and since muscles comprise a large portion of your body weight, learning to let them relax will lead to relaxation of your entire body.

For the first few sessions, you might want to have someone read the technique instructions aloud to you, slowly, one sentence at a time, with ten- to fifteen-second pauses between sentences. Don't worry if you feel foolish and self-conscious at first; you'll get used to it. By the third or fourth session, try doing the technique on your own, as best as you can remember it. Don't be too concerned about precision, or about remembering the exact details of every sequence. Instead, focus on adopting the correct general style.

Basic pointers

In the early weeks of muscle awareness practice, use common sense to avoid unnecessary distractions. For example:

1. Practice without any background noise, such as the radio or stereo.
2. Arrange to have someone answer the phone, if convenient, or unplug it during your session.
3. Don't practice when you're in a hurry.
4. To avoid drowsiness, do not practice in the late evening or right after meals.

It may seem a bit strange that I'm advising against drowsiness during a relaxation exercise. The point of the exercise is not to slip into a sleep pattern but to consciously, and with as much awareness as possible, relax. If you find yourself getting too sleepy, try one or more of the following:

1. Temporarily open your eyes, stretch your arms, and take a couple of deep breaths; then resume the session.
2. Practice in daylight, if possible.
3. Keep the lights on bright, instead of dimming them.
4. Practice in a sitting or semi-reclined position.
5. Vary the sequence of the muscle locations you focus on; for example, proceed from head to toe during one session and from toe to head during the next.
6. Shift your focus from one location to another more quickly than usual, and then repeat the entire sequence a second time.

Preparation

Lie down on your back, with your heels several inches apart and your feet falling naturally to the sides. Let your arms lay away

from your body at a comfortable angle, palms up or down —
whatever feels natural to you. Make any small adjustments
necessary in the positions of your hips, shoulders, neck, and head
until you feel "sunk into the floor" as completely as possible. With
a few days' practice, you'll find this position more naturally and
will automatically get comfortable. Use small pillows under your
neck and lower back if necessary.

Now close your eyes and slowly take a couple of deep breaths.
Begin to focus all your attention on how your breathing feels.
Do not try to control your breathing pattern, but simply become
aware of any or all of the following:

1. The rise and fall of your chest and stomach.

2. The slight stretching and loosening of some chest and rib-
   cage muscles with each breath.

3. The small pause between each exhalation and inhalation.

4. The flow of air into your nose and throat (cool) and back
   out again (warm).

5. How far down into your lungs the air is flowing.

6. Whether the depth of your breathing seems uneven or
   regular.

7. Any other physical aspects of the breathing process that you
   become sensitive to.

After a short time, your breathing will settle into a comfortable, steady, relaxed rhythm, and will no longer be self-
conscious, even though you are observing how it feels. It will
seem to be a physical process that is happening naturally — that
you are conscious of, but not interfering with. Continue this
focus for another moment or so.

Now begin to focus on each of the muscle locations listed
below. Don't move or contract the muscles in order to feel them
better. Don't try to picture them in your mind. Don't recite this
routine to yourself. Don't try to relax the muscles you're focusing on. Don't even "try to feel" the muscles themselves. Simply
direct your attention — focus all your awareness — into each location for a long, quiet moment. If there is any sensation to feel,
you'll feel it without trying.

It does not matter what impression you get of each location
as you focus on it (tense or relaxed, clear or vague, or simply

no impression at all). All that matters is that you quietly and effortlessly focus on each place long enough (several breaths will usually do it) to become aware of it as a location, and to become conscious of any slight or subtle feeling, if there is one.

Don't be concerned about mental distractions or about your mind wandering off to other thoughts. Distractions will always happen, so each time you become aware that you're distracted from the exercise, simply return your attention to the location on which you were last focusing.

The technique

Focus your attention on your right and left calves. Imagine a point deep inside each calf muscle and become conscious of those two locations. Be aware of the pressure of the contact of your calves with the floor. The muscles may feel soft and sunk into the floor, or stiff and pressing against it. This feeling will probably become as clear as it can ever be within the space of several breaths.

Now continue this style of awareness in the following locations – one pair of points or one area at a time – focusing deep inside each muscle:

Arches of feet
Calves
Middle of thighs
Hips and buttocks
Palms of hands
Thick upper portion of forearms
Middle of upper arms
Outside corner of shoulders
Stomach surface, or front abdominal muscles
Chest surface and rib-cage
Lower back muscles
Upper back muscles
Base, back, and sides of neck
Jaw hinges
Cheeks
Eyes
Forehead
Temples
Scalp

Direct your attention to each of these locations every time you do the exercise. Remember, it is not necessary to clearly feel something in every location at every session. The sensations in some muscles can be very subtle. Be patient. The important thing is to direct your attention to each location in turn. It is the method that matters, not the "results." The overall value of this technique (rather than the results of each separate observation) will become clearer to you after you've been practicing it for a couple of weeks. Meanwhile, you will be surprised at how relaxed you are by the end of each session.

Once you've focused on each location, return your attention to your breathing. Become as fully aware of its sensations as you were at the beginning of the session. In addition, become aware of the condition of your four limbs – whether they feel heavy and sinking into the floor, or light and floating, perhaps even missing completely; whether they feel warm or cool, at the skin surface or deep inside; whether they feel tight or loose; and so on.

Next, become conscious of the entire length of your back, from the lower spine to the base of your neck. Be aware of whether your back feels generally stiff and pressed against the floor, or soft and sunk into the floor, as if melted into it. Become conscious of the surfaces of your head and your face – the degree to which they feel blank, slack, drained, empty, and expressionless, like a lifeless mask.

Now, for the next few minutes change nothing at all – no stretching, no deep breathing, no shifting or fidgeting or any other voluntary movement. Leave everything exactly as it is, but let your eyelids open so that you can see the room above and around you.

When you open your eyes, you may feel a little disoriented. The room may seem "dreamlike," or your body may feel "unreal." This is a typical (and harmless) reaction that occurs primarily in the first week or two, especially when the practice has been a good one (clearly felt and deeply relaxing). This moment of total physical passiveness, but with the eyes open, sets a very important example for the brain. It demonstrates that you can think, hear, and even see without the use of any muscles. It shows that you can be completely relaxed physically while remaining mentally aware and attentive. After a week or so of practice, this state will no longer feel strange to you.

Finally, when you feel like it, take a couple of deep breaths, slowly get up, and go about your normal business.

RHYTHMIC BREATHING

Breathing is of great value in relaxation, particularly during the initial stages. It is the only automatic body function that we can consciously control, and by controlling breathing, we can influence all autonomic, and to a certain degree all emotional, responses.

When we are tense and anxious, our breathing pattern becomes shallower and faster, but when we are relaxed it is deeper, slower, and more rhythmical. By practicing breathing in a relaxed way, we can calm our minds and emotions enough to be able to carry on in spite of the stress life hands us. Rhythmic breathing exercises are very simple, and can be done at home or even while waiting in line at the supermarket checkout. Only you will know you are doing them once you become familiar with them.

The technique

Ideally, you should practice rhythmic breathing twice a day for between five and fifteen minutes in a quiet room, free of disturbance. Avoid distractions such as sunlight, a clock, animals, and so on.

Rest on your back with your head and neck comfortably supported, with a pillow under the knees to take the strain off both them and your back. Sitting in a reclining position may suit you better – try both positions. Place your hands on your upper abdomen, close your eyes, and get comfortable.

The aim is to breathe slowly, deeply, and rhythmically. Take a deep breath; inhalation should be slow, unforced, and unhurried. Silently count to four, five, or six as you inhale. When inhalation is complete, exhale through the nose, letting your chest fall naturally and slowly. Again, count to four, five, or six, as when breathing in. *The exhalation should take as long as the inhalation.*

There should be no sense of strain. If at first you feel you have breathed as deeply as you can by the count of three, don't worry. Gradually try to extend the inhalation until a slow count of five or six is possible, with a pause of two or three between inhaling and exhaling.

This pattern of breathing should be repeated fifteen to twenty times and, since each cycle can take up to fifteen seconds, the whole exercise should take a total of about five minutes.

Once the mechanics of this technique have been mastered, introduce thoughts at different parts of the cycle. For example, on inhalation you might try to sense a feeling of warmth and energy entering your body with the air, and on exhalation, you might try to sense a feeling of sinking and settling deeper into the surface that is supporting you.

When you have completed the exercise, do not get up immediately, but rest for a minute or two, allowing your mind to become aware of any sensations of stillness, warmth, heaviness, and so on.

Once mastered, this exercise can be used in any tense situation with the certainty that it will defuse the normal agitated response. It should thus result in a far greater ability to cope with stress.

MUSCLE CONTRACTION

As I've said, much psychological stress is stored in the large muscles of the body. The next relaxation technique is designed to release this stored tension and so stop the messages of stress going from muscle to brain. In this way, the cycle of anxiety and tension can be broken. This exercise differs from the first one we discussed in that it actively releases the tension, rather than allowing the stored tension to ease its way from the body.

Preparation

Either lay down or sit in a reclining chair. Again, avoid distractions and wear clothes that do not constrict. It is best to precede this exercise with a few cycles of rhythmic breathing; then you are ready to begin.

The technique

Starting with the feet, try to sense that the muscles of the area are not actively tense. Then deliberately tighten them, curling the toes under and holding the tension for five or ten seconds. Then tense the muscles even tighter for a further few seconds, before letting all the tension go and enjoying the wonderful feeling of release. Try consciously to register what your relaxed feet feel like, especially in comparison with how they felt when you were tensing them.

Progress to the calf muscles and repeat the exercise in the same way. First sense the state of the muscles, then tense them; hold the tension, and then tense them even more before letting go. Consciously register the sense of relief.

After relaxing the calf muscles, go on to exercise the knees, then the upper legs, thighs, buttocks, back, abdomen, chest, shoulders, arms, hands, neck, head, and face. The precise sequence is irrelevant, as long as all these areas are treated in the same way. There is a slight possibility that tensing will induce cramp. If this occurs, stop tensing that area immediately and go on to the next.

Some areas, such as the abdomen, may need extra attention. The tensing of these muscles can be achieved either by contracting (pulling in the tummy) or by stretching (pushing outwards). This variation in tensing is also applicable to many other muscles of the body.

When you have covered the whole body, complete the exercise with several minutes of unhurried, warm, relaxed tranquillity. Focus on the whole body. Sense it as heavy and content, free of tension or effort. If you like, you can enhance this feeling with a few cycles of deep breathing. Then get up, have a good stretch, and carry on with your daily life.

If you do not find any of the three relaxation exercises we have discussed to your liking, there are many others you can try. But there are also different body-work techniques available that approach the body as a whole, promoting ease and relieving stress. We'll discuss some of these next.

YOGA

Reaping the full benefit of yoga requires years of commitment, practice, and study. Yoga classes are now offered by most local parks and recreation departments and frequently by community colleges. These classes are usually excellent and provide a way to enter a whole new world of stress management through body movement, postures, breathing, and relaxation.

Yoga cannot be faulted as a form of exercise and body integration that relaxes and helps to bring about a sense of inner ease. In the religion and culture from which it stems, yoga is but one step in a whole journey toward spiritual enlightenment.

I will not give any suggestions here as to the positions (asanas) you should use, since yoga should be practiced with the guidance of a good teacher, of which there are now many.

DANCE

There is nothing new about humanity's love affair with dance, but it seems to be reaching new peaks of freedom and expression. Creative dance is a wonderful way to feel and express physical poise, which in turn is an expression of ease and relaxation. It is not the skill but the enjoyment that counts.

It doesn't matter whether you choose ballet or ballroom, disco, ballet or break dancing. It doesn't matter whether you dance with others, dance in formation, dance to music, or dance through the woods. What matters is the sense of release that often comes with this form of movement.

THE ALEXANDER TECHNIQUE

The Alexander technique is a way of becoming more aware of your balance, poise, and movement in everyday activities. This awareness can bring into consciousness sensations of tension that were previously unnoticed, and so helps us differentiate between the tensions and efforts that are necessary for poise and those that aren't.

The Alexander technique is concerned with posture and relaxation – two ideas not usually seen as one – and goes beyond relaxation as something we "do," treating it instead as an attribute of being. Thus the deep relationship between physical and psychological ease can be seen at work in our posture.

Posture is far more complex than just sitting or standing straight. It is the way we support and balance our bodies against the ever-present pull of gravity while we go about our daily lives. A whole array of natural postural reflexes organizes this support and balance without any great effort, provided we have the necessary degree of what has been called "relaxation in activity" to allow these reflexes to work freely.

The mechanisms of support, balance, and poise are very delicate and are easily interfered with. The emotional and physical strains of life can soon become fixed in the body in the form of chronic muscle tensions and patterns of distortion throughout the body. Teachers of the Alexander technique use their hands to gently unravel the distortions and encourage the reflexes to work again. In this way, a balance is found between the degree of muscle tone (tension) needed to support the body against the pull of gravity and the degree of relaxation needed to allow free movement, breathing, circulation, and digestion. In addition, teachers help their clients become conscious of their own patterns of "interference," suggesting ways to change them.

It is best to work with a skilled trainer when learning this technique. Advice on how to find a trainer can be obtained from The American Center for the Alexander Technique, 129 W 67th St, New York, NY 10023 (212 799-0468).

MANIPULATION

The techniques of osteopathy and chiropractic may be helpful in releasing locked-in muscle tension or in relieving structural problems of the skeleton that cause muscular tension. Such work must be undertaken only by a skilled practitioner, in the hands of whom much can be achieved.

TOUCH

Touching is one of the most natural human activities. We touch to comfort, to arouse, and to communicate. A whole range of therapeutic touch techniques have been developed that can be used for anything from gently rubbing a bruise to the skilled release of a lifetime accumulation of chronic muscle tension. These touch-based approaches to healing work holistically in that they view the body and mind as one system. They acknowledge the flow from mind to body that can cause psychosomatic conditions, and also the somatopsychic flow from body to mind.

Some touch-based therapies play an active role in psychotherapeutic body work. The work of Wilhelm Reich and the whole field of bioenergetics fall into this category. However, these therapies go beyond the range of this chapter, in which we are concentrating on techniques for promoting relaxation.

MASSAGE

Massage is a beautiful way to relax. Massage techniques vary from the very physical and extreme manipulations given to football players to the gentle stroking of newborn babies. Good masseurs are worth their weight in gold!

For relaxation, the gentler forms of massage, which release body tension through skilled and caring movements, are best. One of the most powerful things about massage is the intimate physical contact established between the two people involved. We don't often touch in our society, and when we do, it has sexual connotations. Physical sensuality does not mean sexuality. It is an acknowledgment that the body deserves care and attention.

Massage is enhanced if you use the essential oils discussed in the section on aromatherapy. The combined benefit of plant oils and human touch can achieve miracles.

In a book of this kind, it is impossible to teach you the techniques of massage. A number of excellent massage guides that are simple to use and well illustrated are listed in the bibliography.

Shiatsu

Shiatsu is a very specialized form of massage, designed to relieve muscle tension and fatigue through direct pressure. Treatments consist of pressure on a specific sequence of points, designed to affect certain muscle systems. The basis for Shiatsu is in Chinese medicine, which sees the roots of physical disease as energy imbalances in the major systems of the body. One cause of energy blockage is muscular tension, and alleviating the tension brings back normal functioning.

EXERCISE

Any gentle exercise will have a toning effect on the body and will bring with it a sense of relaxation. Some physically inclined people take exercise to the point of exhaustion. This goes beyond relaxation and can actually become another stress on the body.

Healthy exercise of some form should be part of any stress management program, from gentle country walks all the way through jogging to hard-core aerobics. Choose what suits you. Being at ease with the process is always the clue to what is best.

SEVEN

Psychological Techniques

Recent years have seen great advances in the understanding of the mind and emotions. Along the way, many techniques have sprung up to enable us to recognize and heal the hurts and pains that accrue through life. We will not look at them all here, as this book deals primarily with the way in which herbs can help alleviate stress and anxiety, but some of them offer useful insights that are worth examining.

Any attempt to ease the impact of stress or soothe the anxieties of life must focus not only on our physical bodies but also on our attitudes, expectations, assumptions, and general perceptions of life. The way we feel is created by what has been called our "mind set," which is the context of thoughts and beliefs that accumulate from the cradle to the grave. Our mind set is approachable and changeable; we can "change our minds."

Many of the techniques that have been developed to facilitate psychological transformation are worthy of books of their own. In fact a whole library could be filled with the theories and techniques that have been developed. In this section, I will briefly touch on the role of the psychological techniques, and then give some examples and self-help contacts.

PSYCHOTHERAPY (COUNSELING)

Psychotherapy is a discipline that involves communication between a client and a therapist. It can take many forms, depending on the therapist's theoretical orientation, the client's problems, and the goals of the treatment. Despite the great range of approaches, a common characteristic is that they all make use of an interpersonal relationship in which the therapist communicates to the client that he or she understands, respects, and wants to help. Other features are the development of a rationale, or "myth," that explains the distress and previous methods of dealing with it, the exploration of the source of the problem, and the exploration of possible alternatives that might lead to a solution. Usually self-esteem is boosted, and the experience of success and of feeling good is fostered. Importantly, psychotherapy is conducted in a locale designed as a place of healing.

Psychotherapy techniques are sometimes divided into two simple, but somewhat misleading, classifications: those that are essentially supportive in aim, and those that seek to obtain a much deeper understanding of the person's past and present in order to bring about therapeutic changes. We'll use these two classifications here, but bear in mind that they are far from mutually exclusive. Insight therapies such as psychoanalysis or psychosynthesis, can be very supportive, while a supportive relationship can help bring about insights and changes.

Supportive psychotherapy

Supportive psychotherapy is intended to offer support during a difficult period. By seeing a therapist at regular intervals during such a time, we may be able to talk through fears and worries and thus find a way of handling our difficulties. The technique is basically palliative and primarily intended to relieve distress. Regular contact with an accepting "authority" figure and the opportunity to discuss problems may lead to positive changes, such as the restoration or strengthening of coping behaviors that may have been impaired by the stressful situation. The role of the therapist is that of the accepting, empathic listener, who encourages us to talk and to express emotions, and who helps us deal with guilt, shame, or anxiety. Relatively little training may be necessary to practice this kind of psychotherapy, since the emphasis is more on listening than on skillful guidance or treatment.

Supportive psychotherapy is particularly valuable when extreme stress gives rise to intense worry or anxiety, and it tends to be most effective when the client's personality is basically sound and the stressful situation is short lived. Most medical herbalists, as well as most family doctors, probably consider offering this kind of support one of their primary roles in our stressful times.

Insight Psychotherapies

It is more difficult to summarize the aims and techniques of the "insight," or "reconstructive," therapies, which are concerned with giving clients increased self-understanding and bringing about changes in attitudes, goals, and emotional responses. The techniques range from the analytical approach of classical psychoanalysis to newer therapies based on a spiritually integrated view of humanity. Such therapies must be conducted by skilled practitioners and involve a degree of commitment and motivation on the part of the clients.

AUTOGENIC TRAINING

Although autogenic training (AT) is a relaxation therapy, I have included it here, under "Psychological Techniques," because it works through psychological pathways. It is a highly systematized technique designed to generate a state of "psychophysiologic relaxation"—a physical state completely opposite to the one that occurs under stress. Through the generation of this state, called the autogenic (self-generated) state, recuperative and self-healing processes are brought into play, presumably through its effects on the autonomic nervous system. This technique forms the foundation for the more inclusive system known as autogenic therapy.

The standard exercises

Six standard exercises form the foundation of autogenic training. These exercises are taught in a very structured fashion. Following the completion of a detailed medical/psychological history, the trainee is shown how to assume a specific training posture (intended to reduce to a minimum any distracting stimuli), how to do a particular exercise, and how to end the exercise. The trainee then practices these techniques for several

Table 3: The six standard autogenic training exercises

Standard exercise	Physiological state	Phrase
1.	Heavy extremities	"My arms and legs are heavy."
2.	Warm extremities	"My arms and legs are warm."
3.	Calm and regular heartbeat	"My heart is calm and regular."
4.	Calm and regular breathing	"My breathing is calm and regular."
5.	Warm solar plexus	"My solar plexus is warm."
6.	Cool forehead	"My forehead is cool."

minutes at least three times a day, and keeps a log of any experiences. The trainer monitors the trainee's progress and determines from observation and from the log entries whether the trainee is ready to move on to the next exercise.

Each exercise involves the use of a specific phrase intended to generate a particular physiological state. While practicing, the trainee is instructed to "attend" passively to a particular part of the body while mentally repeating one of the phrases. For example, the first exercise is concerned with the generation of heaviness in the extremities. The trainee begins by passively attending to the dominant arm and mentally repeating several times, "My right (left) arm is heavy." After focusing on this arm, the next step is to generalize the heaviness to all limbs ("My left (right) arm is heavy"; "Both arms are heavy"; "My arms and legs are heavy") before moving on to the next exercise. The six exercises are summarized in Table 3.

The adjunctive techniques

AT has four so-called adjunctive techniques: autogenic modification, autogenic neutralization, autogenic meditation, and interdisciplinary techniques. We will look at only the first three here.

Autogenic modification uses the autogenic state as a way of bringing about specific changes. This approach involves using a phrase, in addition to or in combination with the standard exercises, that focuses either on physiological change or on attitudinal/behavioral change. For example, a trainee with chronic constipation might add the phrase, "My lower abdomen is warm" to the standard exercises in order to stimulate movement of the bowels. The phrase "Breath carries the words" might be used by a stutterer, and "I am satiated" by an obese person.

Autogenic neutralization allows the carefully supported release of feelings in order to neutralize or reduce their disturbing effects. The trainee is encouraged to talk about either material related to a theme or whatever comes to mind. Of crucial importance in the practice of this technique is the maintenance of an attitude of passive acceptance by both trainee and trainer, so that any sensations that come up are neither suppressed nor enhanced.

Autogenic meditation consists of a series of seven exercises begun only after the trainee has developed the ability to maintain passive concentration for at least thirty minutes (usually after at least six months of AT practice). The focus of the exercises progresses from color, concrete objects and images, feelings, and people to a state where the trainee directly poses questions to the unconscious.

DESENSITIZATION

Relaxation is all very well for those rare times when it is convenient to go through the techniques we discussed earlier. When it's not convenient, however, you will need to use other approaches to desensitize yourself to a particularly problematic situation – in other words, to actually change the way you react to the world. Much good counseling aims at this, but there is a simple way to start the process yourself.

A good first step is to take a sheet of paper, sit down for a few minutes, and write out a list of people, places, activities, and circumstances that you know produce tension in you. You should include only those items that come up regularly in your daily or weekly life. Some possible examples include:

Dealing with your spouse.

Dealing with an in-law.

Dealing with your own parents.

Dealing with your own children.

Dealing with any children (a good one for teachers!).

Dealing with or just facing your boss.

Meeting deadlines.

Making an important decision.

Giving speeches or oral reports.

Taking a test or exam.

Competing, at work or games.

Driving in heavy traffic.

Driving long distances.

Being in a crowded room.

Being in a very small space.

Being in a wide open space.

Looking down from a height.

Waking up/getting up in the morning.

Visiting a doctor.

Visiting a dentist.

Taking pills.

Cooking, cleaning, or other housework.

Typing or other desk work (writing a book!).

Doing your taxes.

Being in an elevator.

Dealing with other people, places, activities, or situations.

Include in your list only those things that cause a distinct physical tension or anxiety response in you. Some may provoke very strong reactions; others may have a lot milder effect on you. But they all should be things that come up regularly or at least periodically.

Keep this list with you, and for the next week or so, when you notice yourself tensing up over something, make sure that "something" is on your list. As soon as your list has at least half a dozen entries, you can begin the process of desensitization and start learning to be at ease with the things that now make you tense.

In order for desensitization to work, you must practice it consistently for a few weeks, but without impatiently expecting dramatic results. Remember, your stress reactions became ingrained in you over a long period of time. A lot of your physical tension is an unconscious habit by now, and is not reversible overnight. As when learning any new skill – or when unlearning any bad habit – it takes a while to alter behavior patterns, and you will succeed only with regular practice.

The technique

First look at your list. Choose an item that has a moderate stress-producing effect on you (not the strongest tension producer and not the weakest). Let it be something that comes up pretty often, say more than once a week, and if possible, choose something that occurs at specific, predictable times – this makes it much easier to prepare for.

No matter what the trigger is, you can learn to be at ease in a recurring stressful situation by taking the following steps.

First do a complete relaxation exercise. When you are feeling deeply relaxed, start to imagine clearly the situation that causes you distress. Visualize with as much depth and clarity as possible the physical situation and people involved. Start at the beginning of the situation and run through in your imagination the series of events as they would normally occur. If at any time in the exercise you actually respond with muscular tension or breathing changes, stop visualizing for a moment and instead, focus on your breathing, be aware of your muscles, and allow yourself to sink back into a relaxed state. Only then should you continue visualizing where you left off. Each time you feel any physical tension at all, let go of your mental pictures, regain the calm state, and breathe more deeply with each exhalation.

The next step is to use your awareness when out in the world but not in the particular situation that causes you stress. Take a few moments to do some breathing exercises so that you become relaxed but poised. Imagine the stressful situation while also feeling this poise. Repeat these exercises more and more often as the time for the stressful situation to occur approaches. They will prepare and desensitize you to the trauma you have come to associate with the situation, and will train your body to remain relaxed in the very situations you would usually brace yourself for. You can thus learn to be responsible and concerned without having to suffer physical symptoms as a result.

After a week or so, the first target of desensitization will probably cause you less tension. You can then choose another from your list and repeat the process all over again. You will find that with each new target, you find it easier and quicker to relax. Not only will you learn to deal with specific situations, you will also acquire the general skill of physical relaxation. Most important, you will enjoy yourself more, as you become calmer and more in control of your life and your reactions to it.

SOCIAL SUPPORT

Many of the stresses that assail us are compounded by feelings of helplessness. Perhaps people were once able to cope with anything that came their way, but today life has become far too complex. Our problems can seem almost insurmountable when we feel isolated, with no one to turn to. It is at these times that other people can be so important. They can, of course, provide useful advice, but much more important is the experience of shared human feeling, support, and understanding.

I am not talking here about the excellent but rather cumbersome official agencies, but about the growing number of self-help and support groups that are now in existence. They are a wonderful expression of the care and compassion that people show for each other when the need arises. A selection of these groups, with addresses and sometimes a brief description of their work, is given below. It is not a comprehensive list but provides a place to start looking for a group or agency that will be able to help you. By providing this list, I am not suggesting that you ignore the help offered by the "Welfare State" in all its forms. Although the system has its problems, it is often run by caring and skilled people. Social services departments, public health centers, and other agencies are there to provide help and support. They can also refer you to other public and private agencies that might better suit your needs.

American Association for Marriage and Family Therapy
1717 K St, Suite 407, Washington, DC 20006 (202 429-1825)
   The oldest organization of its kind in the US, with divisions throughout the country.

Jewish Board of Family and Childrens Services
120 W. 57 St, New York, NY 10019 (212 582-9100)

Consultation Service of the Archdiocese of NY
1011 1st Ave, New York, NY 10022 (212 371-1000)

Parents Without Partners
7910 Woodmont Ave, Suite 1008, Bethesda, MD 20813 (301 654-8850)
   A nationwide organization that provides support for single parents. There are self-help groups throughout the country.

Greater NY Fund United Way
99 Park Ave, New York, NY 10016 (212 557-1050)

The Compassionate Friends
PO Box 1347, Oak Brook, IL 60521 (312 323-5010)
   An organization of bereaved parents who seek to help other bereaved parents by giving them the opportunity to speak freely to an understanding and compassionate friend.

American Association of Retired Persons
1909 K St NW, Washington, DC 20049 (202 728-4888)
   Includes a support program for widows and a women's initiative department.

National Institute of Mental Health
50600 Fishes Lane, Rockville, MD 20857 (301 443-4513)

National Depressive and Manic Depressive Association
Merchandise Mart, PO Box 3395, Chicago, IL 60654 (312 446-9009)

Samaritans USA
PO Box 480, Falmouth, MA 02540 (617 548-8900)

National Organization for Women
1401 New York Ave NW, Washington, DC 20005-2102 (202 347-2279)

Parents Anonymous Inc.
22330 Harthorne Blvd, Suite 208, Torrance, CA 90505 (213 371-3501)

National Self-Help Clearing House
33 W 42nd St, New York, NY 10036 (212 840-1259)

American Cancer Society
Your local chapter will be listed in the Yellow Pages for your area.

Alcoholics Anonymous
468 Park Ave S, New York, NY 10016 (212 686-1100)
A world-wide voluntary fellowship of people whose aim, mutually reinforced, is to attain and maintain sobriety. There are no fees, the only requirement for membership being the desire to stop drinking. The program is one of total abstinence, based on staying away from alcohol one day at a time. A local AA phone number can be found in most telephone directories.

Al-Anon
1372 Broadway, New York, NY 10018 (212 302-7240)
An organization that helps relatives and friends of problem drinkers, whether or not the drinker seeks help or even recognizes the need to do so. Anonymity is strictly preserved.

Narcotics Anonymous
PO Box 622, Sun Valley, CA 91352 (213 764-4880)

EIGHT

Spiritual Integration

All the techniques for achieving a state of inner ease that we've discussed so far have focused on the world around us and our relationship with it. Herbs are seen as gifts from our world to ease our path through life; relaxation and massage are ways of soothing a tense and troubled body; and psychotherapy quiets the storm of emotions that tends to drown us at times. There is, however, another way to approach stress, a way that starts from within, at our very core.

There is a spiritual, ineffable center to all human life and to all motivation and action. This spiritual center, whether we call it the soul, God, the life force, or whatever, is the foundation of our individual lives, the light that illuminates, and the source of inner healing and ease. We could say God is the best remedy for stress!

There are many paths to the spirit. Religion is the path chosen by many people, and a committed Christian, Jew, Moslem, or Buddhist may view their belief systems as a door through which meaning, spiritual love, and indeed God are reachable. However, the spirit is freely available to all of us, no matter what our beliefs. Moreover, meditation and other methods of attaining inner peace do not compromise those beliefs. Christians can meditate without denying their faith, and so can Jews. In the West, meditation has an Eastern "occult" aura about it that is ridiculous and unfounded. In this section we will consider meditation along with other techniques as ways to ease tension by achieving spiritual poise.

LOVE AND PURPOSE

Today, many people are profoundly uneasy not only with their own lives but also with the direction in which our whole society is moving. We are bombarded with stories of ecological crisis, economic collapse, and wide-spread starvation, all enveloped in the fear of nuclear megadeath. These massive issues may seem out of the hands of us simple folk, but there is a direct relationship between the stress they cause and the personalized stress that can, for example, cause migraine. We could say that humanity as a whole has migraine at the moment!

I do not mean to put the weight of the planet's ills on each of our shoulders, but to show that there may be more behind our feelings of stress than we are consciously aware of. Our unease is often too deep to be felt for what it is, or too uncomfortable to be spoken of. The result is a dangerous split in our awareness of our own selves, and loss of both the love that is a keynote of being human and the purpose that gives our lives meaning.

To feed the emotional and spiritual starvation we often consider normal, and to permanently "cure" anxiety, tension, and stress, we must experience the soaring potential of who we are. Only when we clear up the "ecological crisis" in our own lives, when we recognize the wisdom of love and the hope that springs from clarity of purpose, will we achieve inner ease. This is not synonymous with outer ease, for the insights gained from spiritual regeneration often prompt much activity in the world. But amidst this activity, we will have found the inner poise that is the well-spring of healing.

PRAYER

A profound and wonderful way of achieving inner peace is through the path of prayer. Prayer is a way of communing with or approaching the spirit. All spiritual paths have their own ways of prayer, and each individual develops his or her own way of praying.

It is worth noting that, in English, the words for prayer and for the person praying – the prayer – are the same. There is a hint here that in a deep and mysterious way we become the path, we become the prayer as we use it.

In this book, I am not going to suggest specific prayers to use or ways to pray; rather I will simply remind you that inner ease is a gift that comes with selfless prayer.

SPIRITUAL HEALING

The spirit acts directly upon us but it can also be "directed" or invoked by a spiritual healer. As a book on herbal remedies for stress, this is not the place to explore this deep and profound realm; but this section would not be complete without mention of the excellent work done by some spiritual healers. While many are nonprofessionals, a basic duty of the ministers of the Church is healing the sick. Not all priests feel at ease with this work, but in times of stress, the Church can, for some people, be a haven of peace and healing.

MEDITATION

Whenever we focus our attention on something, we are meditating. Whether we are a "captain of industry," a gardener, or a Zen monk, the difference is only the degree to which we are focusing and the purpose of the whole exercise. Meditation can be a profound and powerful tool in the expansion of consciousness and the exploration of the spirit; however, it is just as relevant as a gentle way of reducing stress and moving to a place of ease and inner poise.

The term *meditation* covers a whole spectrum of approaches and techniques. In the West, in these days of crisis and transformation, we are fortunate indeed to have increasingly more of the spiritual wisdom and skill of the East available to us. A plethora of teachers, schools, and books is ready to help us explore the more profound depths of meditation. The techniques described below may well whet your appetite for more. Don't hesitate to take the plunge!

Levels of meditation

Western medical research has focused on meditation as a way to gain control – as a "self-regulation strategy." This research initially investigated the physiological changes that consistently occur during meditation, including a reduction in the heart rate, a decrease in bodily oxygen consumption, a lowering of the blood pressure, an increase in skin resistance, and an increase in the regularity and strength of alpha activity in the brain. Because these qualities indicate a state of quietness in the autonomic nervous system, doctors suggested that meditation would be a useful self-regulation technique for relaxation training.

Not surprisingly, clinical research has borne this out. In a recent academic review of the psychotherapeutic and health-related effects of meditation, its value was shown in:

1. Reducing stress and tension. Meditators give subjective reports of decreased feelings of stress and anxiety, as well as objective physiological indications of stress reduction.

2. Decreasing addictive behaviors. In studies of addiction, meditators consistently report a larger reduction in usage than non-meditators, for drugs ranging from alcohol and marijuana to LSD and heroin.

3. Lowering blood pressure. The research consistently shows a reduction in blood pressure in meditators, a reduction in the use of medication, and a reduction of bodily symptoms.

This scientific appraisal of meditation also shows how the therapist is changed by the process of healing or helping. Therapists using meditation in their work report that it helps them become more open and receptive to their clients' concerns.

Most research in the West has been carried out in laboratories and other settings that used relatively short-term meditators as subjects. Remember, however, that meditation originally evolved within the philosophical-religious context of the Eastern spiritual disciplines. It was a technique used primarily as a means of inducing altered states of consciousness, changing a person's ordinary perception of the world, and developing a more intimate, unified, and accepting view of oneself, of nature, and of other people.

There can be no doubt that, when used in this way, profound changes can occur during meditation. These can range from slight alterations in perception in short-term meditators to more profound experiences. The following descriptions of their experiences from meditators give a taste of the possibilities: "self-transcendence"; "felt meaning in the world"; "a heightened sense of connectedness with the world and with others, a sense of purpose and meaning"; "deep positive emotion."

These very powerful inner experiences have obvious implications for health, because they influence the way we relate not only to ourselves but also to other people and to the world around us. Just as important are the social implications, as people who use meditation in this way transform themselves and their approach to life. It is one of the signs of hope for the future that a growing number of people meditate and are willing to put into practice the reappraisal it brings about.

There are hundreds of techniques that could be called meditation. The practices used to bring about the meditative state are as diverse as gazing quietly at a candle flame, concentrating on the mental repetition of a sound or mantra, following one's own breathing, concentrating on the imagined sound of rainfall, chanting a ritual word or phrase out loud, attending to body sensations, passively witnessing the flow of thoughts through the mind, concentrating on an unanswerable riddle, or whirling around in a dance. The aim is always the same – to alter the way the meditator experiences his or her own existence. What follows is a simple guide to basic types of meditation and how to use them in practice.

Basic pointers

Meditation will only be effective in stress reduction or spiritual development if you are properly prepared and in a receptive frame of mind. Here are some basic pointers for preparation. You will notice similarities between these suggestions and those for preparing for relaxation exercises.

1. Don't meditate within an hour after eating a meal. The meditative traditions insist that meditation is ineffective on a full stomach. Coffee, tea, and other caffeine-containing drinks, such as Coca-Cola, should be avoided. The need to avoid stimulants should be obvious: meditation is for calming down.

2. Choose a quiet room to meditate in, where you can be alone. If someone else is present, he or she should be meditating as well. Unplug the phone or take it off the hook. Let others in the house know you are meditating and that you would ap-

preciate stillness. Shut pets out of the room in case they disturb you. It can be quite a shock to have a cat jump on your lap when meditating!

3. Face away from any direct light, and though the room need not be dark, it is more pleasant if the lighting is subdued.

4. Sit in a comfortable, easy position on a straight-backed chair or on a cushion on the floor. (It is best to have your back straight.) It will help to loosen tight clothes and remove shoes.

5. If during meditation you become uncomfortable, change your position slightly, stretch, yawn, or scratch. When using meditation for stress reduction, the point is to be at ease, not to discipline yourself like a Zen monk, who focuses on mastering distractions and not necessarily being at ease.

6. If you are interrupted, try not to suddenly jump up out of meditation. You are likely to be in a deeply relaxed state, so gently and slowly stretch and then get up. Ideally, return to meditation afterwards.

7. The length of a meditation session is up to you. The times suggested for each technique may not feel comfortable at first. Take as long or as short a time as you like.

8. If you find that meditation suits you, schedule sessions into your life so that they become a regular daily routine. Occasional use of the technique, while pleasant, will not bring about any lasting benefits. It is best to meditate twice a day, but you should try to do so at least once daily.

9. Approach meditation with a gentle, non-forcing attitude. The techniques described below should not prove difficult even for those unfamiliar with them. Don't try to do the meditation exercises "correctly," but instead let each meditation session "do" itself. There is no "good" and "bad" here.

10. Meditating to aid stress reduction does not involve focusing the mind. Whenever thoughts enter (and they often will), simply treat them as you might clouds drifting across the sky. Don't try to push them away or hold on to them, simply watch them come and go. When you realize that your mind is caught up in thoughts, gently come back to your object of focus with-

out forcing. Extraneous thoughts are a natural part of the meditative process.

11. After finishing a session, remain seated for a moment or two with your eyes closed. During this time, allow your mind to return to everyday thoughts. This helps to carry the tranquillity achieved during the session into your daily life. Then, very slowly, open your eyes and get up.

The mantra technique

Mantra or sound meditation uses a word or syllable as a focus for concentration. Three suggestions are Ah-nam, Ra-ma, and Peace, or you can use a word of your own. When choosing your mantra, first repeat each of the words you are considering (either mentally or out loud) and then select the one that sounds the most pleasant and soothing. Avoid using a word that is emotionally "loaded": no names of people; no words that bring too intense or exciting an image. Your mantra should ring in your mind and bring a sense of serenity. Before you tell someone else which mantra you have chosen, ensure that they understand that regardless of how they feel about it, your mantra is to be respected. It will come to have a special meaning for you and will become a signal to turn inward toward a peaceful state.

Having selected your mantra, sit in a comfortable position. With your eyes open and resting on a pleasant object, such as a plant, say the mantra out loud to yourself, repeating it slowly and rhythmically. Experiment with the sound; play with it. Then as you repeat the mantra, say it more and more softly, until it finally becomes a whisper.

Now stop saying it out loud, close your eyes, and simply listen to the mantra in your mind. Let your facial muscles relax and think the mantra but do not say it.

That is all there is to mantra-meditating: sitting peacefully, hearing the mantra in your mind, allowing it to change any way it wants – to get louder or softer; to disappear or return; to stretch out or to speed up. Meditation is like drifting on a stream in a boat without oars – you don't need oars because you are not going anywhere.

Continue meditating for fifteen minutes. When the time is up, just sit quietly without meditating for another two to three minutes.

The breathing technique

Several ancient and powerful meditation techniques focus on the breath. They are not primarily aimed at relaxation, but at personal and spiritual transformation. The guidelines here are very basic and are designed to aid the relaxation process.

Sit in a comfortable position and take a single slow, deep breath, saying to yourself the word "in" as you breathe in, and the word "out" as you breathe out. After taking this first deep breath, do not intentionally influence your breathing. Let your breathing go its own way, fast or slow, shallow or deep – whatever way it wishes. As it does so, say to yourself "in" as you inhale and "out" as you exhale.

After a while, try to extend the sound in your mind so that at all points in the meditation you are either thinking "in...n...n...n" or "ouuuuuuut...t...t" in long, easy sounds. Meditate naturally, with no concern about doing it correctly. If you skip an "in" or "out" because your mind has wandered (as it will), you can always pick up the words whenever you are ready.

If the words fade and you find you are just sensing your breath, that's fine. It means you have quieted down.

When fifteen minutes are up, come out of meditation gradually and gently.

The visual technique

To practice visual meditation, first select a pleasant natural object, such as a plant, flower, piece of fruit, bit of driftwood, or an object like a simple vase. Although a candle flame is sometimes used for visual meditation, it is not suggested here because if not properly used, its glare may cause eye strain.

Place your chosen object on a table at or near eye level and at a distance of two to four feet from you. Adjust this distance to the most comfortable focus for your eyes and eliminate distracting objects in the immediate background.

Sit comfortably and allow your eyes to come to rest on the object, but do not try to see it. Make no effort to focus. Instead, allow the object to come into your vision – let it enter your awareness. Do not make any conscious attempt to think about it in any way – what it is, what it means, its name, the class of objects it belongs to – but don't worry if such thoughts come to your mind spontaneously. Just look at your object innocently, as a child might.

Avoid staring, for this can cause eye strain. During this meditation, your eyes will want to move about, spontaneously traveling over the object. Allow them to. Do not stop your eye movements; they are part of "seeing."

Because most of us can only look at things with "the eye of the beginner" for a few seconds at a time, this meditation consists of a series of new beginnings. After allowing the object to remain in your field of vision for about seven to ten seconds (this interval may be longer or shorter depending upon your own inclinations), purposely shift your focus to a more distant place in the room. At this time, you can remove your attention from the object and let it wander where it will. Continue gazing away from the object for a few seconds (you will "feel" the right length of time for this part of the process) and then, when you are ready, bring your eyes and your attention gently back to the object. Allow yourself to become absorbed in the object once more (again, for about seven to ten seconds) and then purposely focus elsewhere once again.

Continue in this way – looking at the object, looking away from it, and then returning to it refreshed – for five minutes (this is a shorter meditation technique than the others we've discussed). At the end of five minutes, close your eyes for a minute or so and sit quietly.

HERBS AND SPIRITUAL PEACE

It is completely natural for an herbalist to be at home with spiritual matters. While plant remedies are potent medicines, the plants from which they are devised are also vital for a healthy world in other ways. Our natural surroundings are important to us. Why do people fill their offices with indoor plants? Of course, because they are aesthetically pleasing; but I would suggest that it is through these aesthetic sensibilities that spirituality maintains our sanity.

To the medieval monks, it was obvious that God, through the simple flowers of the field, had given humanity a gift of healing and peace. Today, we are at last relearning this simple truth. Throughout this book I have tried, where appropriate, to show the ways in which herbal remedies link us to our spiritual selves through our planet, Earth. This connection aligns us with yet greater realms of spirit and light. We are indeed one with the Creator of all things. Let us use our herbal remedies with thankfulness and joy, for their very existence is a demonstration of God's unbounding love for us all.

NINE

Managing Stress-Induced Illnesses

When people are seen as whole beings, and not simply as bodies with minds on top of them, it comes as no surprise that there is a deep association between psychology and physiology. This association has profound implications for all illness, not just stress and anxiety.

It is a demonstration of the inadequacies of our scientific approach to health that people are even thought of in terms of the two words, mind and body. As we have already discussed, there is, in reality, one system that should not be separated. However, since there is no one English term for this system, to talk about it in English, and say what needs to be said, is exceedingly difficult!

It is worth examining how orthodox medicine sees the relationship between mind and body in the development of illness. While no all-encompassing explanation for their association has been put forward, the medical world has considered a number of possible explanations:

1. Some physical illness may be psychological in origin; that is, the bodily disturbance is the result of and caused by the psychological illness.

2. Physical illness may arise as an indirect consequence of a mental disorder, the bodily illness resulting from behavioral disturbances that are secondary to the psychiatric problem.

3. Physical methods of treating mental illness may cause

bodily disease. This is unfortunately all too common with the wide use of drug therapy today.

4. The mental disturbance may be a manifestation of a physical illness, or an adverse effect of its treatment.

5. A mental or emotional problem may be a "purely" psychological response to either the physical illness itself or to the significance that the illness has for the person involved.

This might all sound a bit semantic! These explanations are, however, a way of fitting the relationship of mind and body into a pattern that will enable an orthodox medical practitioner to decide which drugs to use. Should he or she focus on the physical problems or the mental disturbance?

From the perspective of a holistic herbalist, this is an artificial and unnecessary question. To help both body and mind, the whole must be treated as a whole. Thus, not only are remedies that are helpful for specific symptoms needed, but a management plan to help us cope with stress is also necessary. This broader view lessens the impact of stress, helps free us, and hopefully creates the space for healing to take place.

EMOTIONAL AND MENTAL RESPONSES TO PHYSICAL ILLNESS

Any illness occurs within the context of our whole lives and so will affect us psychologically and socially, as well as physically. It might be useful for us to consider ways in which illness itself may produce psychological problems. The difference between this type of problem and a problem that affects the body but arises in the mind is purely one of perspective. Technically, if orthodox doctors consider the primary problem to be in the mind, they label it a psychosomatic problem, but if they consider the root of the problem to be in the body, they label it a somatopsychic problem. The distinction is subtle, as shown here:

$$\text{psyche} \longrightarrow \text{(psychosomatic)} \longrightarrow \text{disease}$$
$$\text{disease} \longrightarrow \text{(somatopsychic)} \longrightarrow \text{psyche}$$

Psychological reactions to physical illness are common and may need some sort of specialized help. This help may come from an orthodox psychiatrist, from a holistic health practitioner, or simply from a friend.

Importance of the Patient's Perception

The lack of knowledge about psychological responses to physical illness that is exhibited by most health practitioners reflects their narrow view of the nature of illness. When the illness is seen in strictly biological terms, the patient's own perception of the problem is ignored. For the patient, there is no difference between the biological process of the disease and the repercussions it has on social life and feelings. In a truly holistic way, they are part and parcel of the whole problem. However, if the doctor ignores psychological reactions in favor of medical pathology, further problems can occur that will interfere with treatment and impede recovery.

Psychological reactions to physical illness vary in type and intensity with no clear point beyond which the reactions can be considered "abnormal." Many are common and understandable reactions to the social disruption and fears generated by illness. While severity and type of illness often affect response, the relationship is not clear-cut. A mild illness may give rise to marked emotional changes in one person, while a life-threatening illness will evoke little or no response in another. One way of accounting for this variation is to look at the patient's perception of the problem. This perception will in turn be affected by personality and experience, the nature of the illness, and the social context. It is worth looking at these in more detail.

Personality and experience

Illness is dealt with in different ways by people with different personalities. For example, the extent to which we experience, remember, and complain about pain can be affected by whether we are naturally "highly strung" or "laid back."

The amount of information we are given about the illness can play a large part in diminishing uncertainty and anxiety about both the illness itself and its treatment.

Previous experience of similar problems may give us the sort of information most needed to reduce anxiety. However, if our information comes from seeing apparently similar but actually more serious symptoms in another person, then very strong but possibly groundless fears may build up.

Our psychological state at the time of the illness will play a great part in the way we perceive its severity. If a gallbladder problem arises during a time when we are anxious about another member of the family, or we are having problems paying the mortgage, the experience of physical illness may be much worse, since it is well known that anxiety lower our pain thresholds.

The nature of the illness

There appears to be no direct relationship between the severity of an illness and the possibility of psychological problems accompanying it. However, the likelihood of psychological problems may be higher if the part of the body with the clinical disorder has particular significance. An obvious example is a hand injury for a pianist. It has been suggested that disabling diseases are more threatening for men, whereas disfiguring diseases are more threatening for women. This does not mean that this correlation is natural. We are all at the mercy of the roles we play and the assumptions we make about what makes us attractive or our lives meaningful. What is socially normal may not always be good or sane. Illness, even when extreme, can be an agent of change and an opportunity to grow beyond previous personal boundaries.

The social context

An illness of any severity may have a greater or lesser impact on us depending upon the social context within which it occurs. We may perceive it very unfavorably if it occurs at a bad time, such as when we are starting a new job, but we may accept it with relief if it helps us avoid an unpleasant social situation, such as exams! The reactions of the people around us will also play a role in determining the ultimate impact. The social context can have a direct effect on the perceived severity of a symptom, and may even cause us to delay seeking medical help.

Psychological Reactions to Illness

People commonly respond psychologically to major illness in one of a few ways: with depression, anxiety, or denial. These responses may even occur in more sensitive people when the illness is apparently minor. The psychological response is unique to the person involved and shouldn't be labeled hypochondriacal.

Depression

Depression is the most common response. Studies have shown that between 20 and 30 percent of all medical patients suffer some degree of depression. This may be relatively mild and seem like a "flattening" of the emotions together with some loss of interest in the outside world, or it may be quite pronounced, with emotional discomfort, withdrawal, and even suicidal feelings.

Depression is often associated with an actual or threatened loss. Illness can involve loss of parts of the body or loss of bodily and social functions. There are direct parallels between such losses – real or imagined – and the psychological effects of bereavement.

Depression most often occurs after the initial stages of an illness, when its full implications become apparent. We may interpret the illness as punishment for something we have or have not done in the past, in which case the depression is commonly colored by feelings of guilt and self-criticism, especially if we consider the "punishment" justified.

A "giving-up" complex commonly develops if the patient feels there is little to live for. This complex is characterized by feelings of helplessness and hopelessness. By helplessness, I mean feelings of impotence and failure, or frustration in getting help from the world and other people. Hopelessness refers to the feeling of no longer being able to cope with problems. This complex is common in a short-lived form and passes away when the situation improves. However, for some people, the complex can persist and radically affect both their response to their current illness and their openness to subsequent illnesses.

Anxiety

The anxiety commonly associated with illness stems partially from the reasonable uncertainty the patient may have about the cause and outcome of the illness. It can be compounded by inadequate information given by doctors as to the nature of the problem and the treatment prescribed. As one doctor has put it, "For the patient, no news is not good news; it is an invitation to fear." An herbalist or other practitioner of holistic medicine should not fall into this trap.

Anxiety usually shows as fear, apprehension, and bodily symptoms. These are most prominent in the early stages of the illness and represent a reasonable reaction to the onset of illness and the related uncertainties. In this situation, we should talk freely of our fears and our medical practitioner should supply clear information. This will not only minimize anxiety but also bring about a better healing response.

Denial

Denial is one way in which we deal with threatening situations and it may even be a necessary and adaptive response to the full physical and psychological impact of an illness. It has a protective function, preventing us from being overwhelmed by anxiety. However, it can go too far when it prevents us from making a realistic assessment of the severity of our symptoms. Thus, denial can be the cause of delay in seeking medical help and so may reduce the chances of a favorable outcome.

DIS-EASE AND STRESS

From this discussion, it should be apparent that illness does not occur in isolation but happens to an individual with a particular personality and in a particular social context. Both personal and social factors play a role in determining the impact of an illness, and the nature of the psychological response can provide considerable insight into the patient's underlying personality.

In the rest of this chapter, we will consider some of the physical diseases in which psychological factors play an indisputable part. From a holistic perspective, these factors are present in all conditions and any approach to health must encompass its mental, emotional, and spiritual aspects as well as the physiological. It is, however, worth looking at those conditions specifically recognized as having psychological components, so that herbal, dietary, and stress-management techniques can be seen at work.

Far more psychological research has been done for conditions such as heart disease than for other problems, such as psoriasis. In the discussion that follows, you will find more information in some sections than others. This does not mean that stress is more involved in some problems than others, but simply that more information about its involvement is available. Guidance about herbal remedies is given for each specific disease, but always in the context of the broader approach to stress and anxiety given elsewhere in the book.

ALLERGIES

The allergic reaction can take different forms but commonly appears as hay fever, an itchy rash, a constantly runny nose, wheezing, and joint pains. Different allergies produce similar symptoms because the body reacts to them in the same way – with the release of a chemical called histamine into the bloodstream.

Cause

An allergy is an abnormally sensitive reaction to a substance in the environment that may not in itself be harmful, but that triggers a reaction in sensitive people. These so-called allergens can be almost anything, but the most common are flower or tree pollen, some foods, household pets, and even house dust.

Times of stress or feelings of anxiety and tension usually increase the severity or frequency of allergy attacks. For some people, emotional upsets may even be the main factor involved.

There is a growing recognition that a whole range of conditions appear to be related to "subclinical" allergies, especially to food additives. This is discussed in the section on hyperactivity.

Treatment

Obviously, the basis of any truly helpful treatment or management of allergic reactions is to stop the exposure to the "thing" that is triggering it. This can be quite easy when the trigger has been identified as a certain food or animal, but often simple avoidance is impossible. The most common treatment is then to use drugs called antihistamines, which suppress the reaction that the allergen is eliciting in the body. For a holistic practitioner, this is a possibly harmful or at least a limited approach, for acupuncture, homeopathy, and even chiropractic have much to contribute toward the alleviation of this complaint.

Herbal remedies

The plant kingdom has been generous in the provision of herbs that help the body cope with allergies. There are three ways to use these herbs to combat an allergy:

1. Use herbal remedies that help the whole person get well. With this approach, not only do we use antiallergy remedies, but we also use those that help any other specific problems we may have, all in the context of ensuring that our health is at its peak. The liver, lungs, kidneys, and skin are especially important.

2. Use herbs in conjunction with an individually worked-out diet (since each person's triggers are unique). Thus, not only will our diet be based on sound ideas of good nutrition but it will also take into account what we must avoid and will compensate for any nutritional losses we have incurred.

3. Use herbs in conjunction with the other techniques explored in this book to help deal with the impact of stress on our lives. To do this, we will have to select the techniques most relevant to us and then set up a routine for applying them in practice.

As I've said, there are a multitude of plants that can help in allergic reactions, partly because of the individual nature of the reactions and symptoms. Herbs that ease the symptoms of hay fever—such as itching eyes, runny nose, and tight chest—are listed below. Consult a complete herbal for more information, as the herbal at the end of this book concentrates on stress-relieving plants.

ELDER FLOWER AND BERRY: All parts of the elder tree seem to have profound medicinal value. In rural Wales, an elder tree was always planted beside a new house. If only this were done in modern housing developments! The leaves and berries are good for sinus catarrh and the itching of the eyes in hay fever. Elderberry wine works as well!

EYEBRIGHT: As its name suggests, this small meadow flower is renowned as an eye remedy. As a wash, it eases discomfort of the eyes.

GARLIC: In addition to being generally good for us, specifically reduces the impact of allergic reactions.

GOLDENROD: One of the best remedies for sinus catarrh, not only that of allergic origin.

GOLDEN SEAL: A specific tonic for the tissues that line the nose, throat, and sinuses; generally valuable in allergies that affect these places.

NETTLES: Apart from being a "weed" with a painful sting, this is a wonderful herb that can reduce allergic tendencies if used regularly.

PEPPERMINT: This common herb often alleviates the general discomfort of an allergy.

A medical herbalist would also call into play herbs that have an action at a deeper level. These can be quite strong and are best used under professional advice. They include:

MA HUANG: A Chinese remedy that is widely used in Western herbalism as well as Western medicine. Works to reduce the chemical reaction in the blood that is the basis of most allergic reactions, and specifically of hay fever and asthma.

ASTHMA

In an asthma attack, the tubes through which air is carried in and out of the lungs become constricted, either because of contractions of the muscles in the walls of the tubes or because of secretion of a sticky mucus in the tubes themselves. This has the effect of making it more and more difficult to get air in and out of the lungs, producing shortness of breath, wheezing, and a cough. The worse the breathlessness, the greater the feeling of anxiety and even panic. This in turn tends to make the attack worse.

Cause

The basic physiological problem associated with asthma is a reversible obstruction of the small airways of the lungs. Knowing this, however, does not tell us exactly what's involved in the physiological process. An all-encompassing cause for asthma has not been found, but a whole range of triggers are known. Attacks can be triggered in different people by allergies, chest infections, irritant gases, smoke, and psychological factors such as stress and anxiety.

Food allergies are a common predisposing factor. They do not always take the form of overt allergies and can confuse things, since taking the food may not actually trigger an attack. The worst culprits are dairy products – cow's milk, butter, and cheese. They are especially implicated in asthma in children who were not breast-fed or who were weaned onto cow's milk in the first nine months of life. Other widely implicated foods include white sugar, candy, and artificial additives of any kind. Any food might be involved in individual cases, though, so specialist help should be sought in tracking down the culprit. There is much that herbal medicine has to offer in the alleviation of allergies but it is best to work with a medical herbalist, whose training includes nutrition and "clinical ecology," as it is now called.

If a chest infection gets out of hand or occurs in a person very prone to asthma, the congestion that develops can trigger an attack. The usual orthodox treatment for chest infection is a course of antibiotics. However, this treatment may itself cause problems, especially in young children who may be prescribed repeated courses. A good medical herbalist can help greatly, not only by clearing up the infection but by strengthening the lungs and increasing bodily resistance.

Dust or any irritating gas may trigger an asthma attack. The gas could be smoke from a fire or even cold air. By far the most common and worst irritant of this kind is tobacco smoke. Unfortunately, asthma attacks can be triggered not only by smoking cigarettes but from just being around smokers. People with asthma should not feel at all reticent about asking smokers to abstain in their presence.

Psychological factors

Stress does not cause asthma, but in most sufferers, it can act as a trigger or can prolong an attack. Usually it is just one of a combination of factors that produces the attack.

It has been suggested that people suffering from asthma may be in conflict with a key person in their lives, commonly a parent, and yet be unable to express their hostile feelings in either words or actions. Because of their excessive self-control, emotional tension is not adequately discharged until an asthmatic attack acts as an unusual pathway for its release. This process has been described as "suppressed crying." In an attack, asthmatics breathe in but are unable to breathe out, and they seem to choke. Then they can't breathe new air in normally, because they can't "let it all out."

The process of "generalization" can also lead to asthmatic attacks that occur in response to a wide range of situations other than the original precipitating one. The understandable anxiety associated with an attack of asthma may itself lead to a learned, automatic response of airway obstruction that occurs in a wide variety of anxiety-provoking situations.

Treatment

Relaxation and stress management are vital to the treatment of asthma. In addition to dietary advice and herbs, interpretative psychotherapy may be useful in helping to deal with stressful emotional problems. Biofeedback techniques have been particularly helpful in keeping the conscious mind in touch with the body processes and so giving the asthma sufferer a degree of control. Breathing exercises can be especially helpful in young people.

Herbal remedies

A whole range of remedies can be used to help the chest and ease asthma. It is beyond the range of this book to deal thoroughly with remedies for the lungs, though I will mention a few. Please refer to a good modern herbal for more information.

GRINDELIA: An excellent herb for easing asthmatic spasms, grindelia is also used for general prevention. It doesn't taste too good!

WILD CHERRY BARK: This pleasant remedy reduces spasms and cough, and acts as a mild relaxant.

ELECAMPANE: An excellent lung herb that helps clear congestion and strengthen the chest if debilitated.

Herbs that ease nervous tension can be used freely, as well

as muscle relaxants. Among many possibilities, it is worth considering:

CRAMP BARK: As well as easing the smooth muscles of the chest, cramp bark also reduces some of the tension leading to coughing and wheezing.

MOTHERWORT: Especially useful because it aids and strengthens the heart, while also easing anxiety.

SCULLCAP: A generally safe and effective relaxing remedy.

VALERIAN: This stronger relaxing remedy can still be used with safety.

WILD LETTUCE: A relaxing nervine that specifically eases tension in the chest and throat.

AUTOIMMUNE DISEASE

Many of the more intransigent and baffling of the medical scourges of today may turn out to be autoimmune in nature. The conditions that may fit in this category range from rheumatoid arthritis to multiple sclerosis to ulcerative colitis to psoriasis. Some people have even suggested that cancer may have an autoimmune basis.

Cause

Autoimmune disease occurs when the body is attacked by its own immune, or defense, system. This immune system is very effective and strong, so when misdirected, it can cause much havoc. The name and nature of the particular disease varies, depending upon which part of the body is under attack. However, the basis of the problem is similar in each case, in that it is mediated by the immune system. This system is still only slightly understood so I will make no attempt to explain it here.

Treatment

Skilled help is always necessary in the treatment of autoimmune disease. Holistic medicine has much to offer in the treatment of these chronic problems, in that it helps the body as a whole to be as well and as integrated as possible. This often involves removing from the diet and the environment things that may act as stressors on the system. These things could range from specific foods to inappropriate relationships.

From the evidence that research is rapidly building up, there can be no doubt that stress has much to answer for in autoimmune conditions. Whether it is as a cause or just an aggravating factor is not really important. What is vitally important is that stress be replaced with ease. This may be achieved through relaxation or, perhaps more importantly, through the finding of a purpose and meaning in life. Maybe this is the key to an understanding of the scourge of autoimmune disease.

BLOOD PRESSURE

Blood pressure is created by the heart pumping the blood around the body. As the heart contracts, the pressure in the arteries increases quite abruptly; as the heart relaxes, the pressure drops to about two-thirds of its peak value. Blood pressure is measured at its highest (the systolic) and lowest (the diastolic) points.

Most people have peaks of high blood pressure that occur several times during the day, but usually these peaks are transient. In people who suffer from high blood pressure, the abnormal level is sustained. There are health risks involved if either the systolic or diastolic pressure is constantly raised.

Cause

Periods of stress in people's lives are often associated with a rise in blood pressure. With most people, the blood pressure returns to normal if the stress is removed, but with some people, this is not the case. If the blood pressure has been very high for a prolonged period, changes can take place in the arteries that result in high blood pressure continuing even after the stress has been reduced or removed.

High blood pressure has effects on other organs of the body. It makes the heart pump harder and so puts it under more strain. This may cause the oxygen supply to the heart to become insufficient, which could produce an angina attack. Hardening and narrowing of the arteries also becomes much more likely with high blood pressure. This may in turn produce heart attacks and, if the high pressure bursts blood vessels and causes brain hemorrage, strokes. In extreme cases, high blood pressure may affect the kidneys to the point of kidney failure. From this litany of ailments, it is clear that high blood pressure is a major health risk that is liable to shorten life expectancy considerably.

Blood pressure may become high without any symptoms at all. It is often discovered during routine medical checkups. It may be heralded by headaches, dizziness, palpitations, or unexplained fatigue. If you have any reason to suspect that you have high blood pressure, it is always wise to consult a qualified practitioner, whether "orthodox" or "alternative" (an unfortunate and increasingly artificial division).

Treatment

The development of high blood pressure probably depends upon a variety of closely related physical, psychological, and environmental factors. The side-effects of drugs designed to reduce blood pressure include depression and other psychological disturbances. This, combined with the possibility that knowledge of the diagnosis may itself provoke anxiety, explains the reticence among doctors to convey details of blood pressure to patients. From the holistic perspective, it is essential that people suffering from high blood pressure not only be informed of the diagnosis but also be intimately involved in the treatment. This is a vital key in holistic medicine: the acknowledgement that the "patient" is truly responsible and that the basis for any fundamental healing will come from changes from within. These changes cannot be brought about by drugs or herbs alone, though both will reduce high blood pressure, but through an honest appraisal of the quality and goals of one's life.

To treat raised blood pressure effectively may involve changes in life-style and diet, as well as taking medicines.

Life-style

To reduce high blood pressure, it is important to learn how to recognize and control stress. Though it may not be the sole cause of high blood pressure, stress may play an important role. Even if stress is not a contributing factor, which is unlikely, reducing it will do nothing but good. A re-evaluation of life-style and life goals may be called for, and this is often far more effective than any medical treatment, whether herbal, homeopathic, or chemical. Relaxation exercises and possibly meditation have a lot to offer, if the right technique is found. Psychotherapy and counseling can also be of great value for those people who are willing and able to benefit from insight into their lives.

Diet

Diet commonly plays a part in the elevation of blood pressure. The broad approach described later for heart problems should be the basis for a diet to combat or prevent high blood pressure, with some specific additional suggestions. Salt should be completely avoided; it should not be used in cooking or added to food once it is on the table. Milk, butter, and cheese may contribute to high blood pressure and it is worth cutting them out of the diet completely for at least one month, to see if there is a change in the condition. This change will show up not only in blood pressure readings, but also as an improvement in the general state of well-being. Oily foods and fats should be avoided.

Herbal remedies

Because high blood pressure can be caused by a whole range of factors – from stress to kidney failure – many herbs can be used with benefit. A number of remedies play quite specific roles in the normalizing of blood pressure, and two that always come to mind are:

HAWTHORN BERRIES: This wonderful remedy tones up the vessels of the whole circulatory system. It has an action that normalizes blood pressure, never reducing it below normal.

LIME BLOSSOM: The flowers of this beautiful tree work as a gentle relaxant for all stress-related problems, but especially those affecting the heart and blood vessels.

Water retention – real or suspected – may be an associated symptom, in which case gentle herbal diuretics have a role to play:

DANDELION LEAVES: Nature's best diuretic. Whenever we take medication to help rid the body of water, we should be sure to take a supplement of potassium; otherwise there may be a potentially dangerous depletion of this vital mineral. Dandelion leaves get rid of excess water, but provide the body with a net increase in potassium. Nature does indeed look after us!

YARROW: This diuretic is particularly useful for the circulatory system.

A wealth of herbs that help relieve both psychological and physical tension are available to us. The following is but a partial list of the herbs that could be used. It is worth emphasizing again that the relaxants described here are no substitute for the development of a more relaxed, less stressed approach to life. The key is to be at ease.

CRAMP BARK: A useful relaxing remedy for muscle and body tension accompanying a rise in blood pressure. Also makes a good external lotion.

MOTHERWORT: Apart from its other uses, motherwort helps when nervous tension and palpitations accompany high blood pressure.

SCULLCAP: A relaxing nervine with wide applications.

VALERIAN: A strong relaxing remedy that calms and eases the tension common with this condition, and also helps with sleeplessness.

WOOD BETONY: Especially helpful when there is accompanying headache caused by the rise in blood pressure.

THE DIGESTIVE SYSTEM

The whole process of eating and assimilating food is notoriously prone to stress-related problems. Herbal medicine is especially relevant and powerful for the digestive system. We experience a whole range of digestive problems, but many have causes in common. We'll look at only a few specific diseases here.

PEPTIC ULCER

Peptic ulcers are breaches or defects in the lining of the upper part of the digestive tract. They can occur in the first part of the small intestine (duodenal ulcers), in the stomach (gastric ulcers), or in the esophagus (esophageal ulcers). By far the most common symptom of all these ulcers is pain followed by heartburn.

Many people with gastric ulcers find that food aggravates their pain, while those with duodenal ulcers often find their pain is relieved by eating and is brought on by hunger. In both cases, the pain is almost always eased by milk or antacids. However, it is not unusual for someone to have these "typical" symptoms without having an ulcer at all.

Cause

The origin of peptic ulcers is surprisingly complex and somewhat puzzling, and appears to be different for each type of ulcer, though the strong acid in the stomach plays a leading role. The stomach normally produces this strong acid to aid digestion, but protects itself from the acid by secreting mucus to coat its own walls. Food neutralizes the acid, but when the stomach is empty, during periods of stressful work the acid begins to damage the lining of the stomach and starts ulcer formation.

Alcohol, and particularly hard liquor drunk on an empty stomach, will further damage the stomach lining. Smoking will affect the stomach in at least two ways: by increasing acid formation and interfering with the secretion of mucus, and by irritating the lining with tiny amounts of swallowed tar and nicotine. Smoking will thus contribute to ulcer formation and slow down its healing.

A number of drugs will aggravate or even cause stomach ulceration. The most common problem relates to aspirin and the anti-inflammatory drugs used in arthritis. As a general guideline, anyone suffering from indigestion or other stomach problems should avoid anything that contains aspirin or any drug that contains the word salicylf- in the name of its components. It's worth pointing out that originally this group of chemicals was extracted from the bark of willow. The Latin genus name is Salix and hence the chemical's name salicylic acid. Willow bark, however, does not cause the problems just mentioned.

Psychological factors may influence the workings of the stomach, either directly through the vagus nerve (the stomach nerve) or through hormones and other biochemical factors. The effects of mood on gastric-acid secretion are clear. People with duodenal ulcers tend to respond to the sight and smell of food with greater acid secretion than do others. There is no doubt that stress, anxiety, and depression are all pivotal in these digestive conditions.

Treatment

Successful ulcer management must take into account stress, anxiety, and depression as well as purely physical factors. While psychological factors may not be paramount in the cause of ulceration, there can be no doubt that paying attention to them will speed remission and reduce the likelihood of relapse. Bed rest is valuable not only because it leads to a reduction of gastric-acid secretion, but also because it allows the person with the ulcer to get away from a stressful environment. Insight psychotherapy may also have a lot to offer in helping the review and re-evaluation of life-style and life purpose. At the very least, the use of relaxation techniques to foster ease will greatly soften the impact of the problem.

Diet

The best dietary advice for people with peptic ulcers is to avoid anything that will act as an irritant, whether chemical or physical.

Chemical irritants include acid foods, such as vinegar and pickles, any form of alcohol, smoking, fried and roasted foods, carbonated drinks, rich sauces, and sweet foods. These will all increase the impact of the stomach acid on the stomach lining and so aggravate the ulcer.

Physical irritants include too much roughage and extremes of temperature. Even though the virtues of a high-fiber diet are unquestionable, fiber can rub like sandpaper on a peptic ulcer. When an active ulcer is present, it is best to stick to a low- or medium-fiber diet. Any drink or food that is too hot or too cold will also irritate and cause pain.

Herbal remedies

Herbal remedies have a lot to offer in the healing of stomach and digestive ailments. The basis of treatment is initially to calm down irritation and then to promote the healing of any damaged tissue. A wealth of herbs is available, each of which acts in a slightly different way. The following are examples:

COMFREY ROOT: A soothing remedy rich in mucilage. Also

contains the chemical allantoin, which stimulates the healing of wounds. This is the basis of its reputation as the paramount wound herb.

MARSHMALLOW ROOT: Another soothing remedy, rich in mucilage, that coats the ulcer and calms down any inflammation present.

MEADOWSWEET: This natural antacid reduces the impact of excess acid formation in the stomach.

SLIPPERY ELM: This powder is one of the best soothing remedies.

Other remedies that may prove useful are sweet flag, licorice root, Irish moss, and Iceland moss.

As I've already pointed out, anxiety and tension have a direct impact on the stomach and on digestion in general. The following nervine herbs have a lot to offer in the way of calming action:

PEPPERMINT: The whole peppermint family (the Labiates) is especially useful. Also contains aromatic oils that settle the digestive system.

CHAMOMILE: This gentle relaxing nervine eases tension and, at the same time, acts as an anti-inflammatory herb. It is applicable for all nervous problems of digestion.

LEMON BALM: A wonderfully gentle relaxing herb that is quite safe to use regularly. Also relieves wind and some sorts of indigestion.

VALERIAN: This stronger relaxing nervine contains a potent (though unpleasant) oil that also helps settle wind and indigestion.

Other relaxing herbs that can help are scullcap, St. John's wort, pasque flower, hops, and passionflower.

IRRITABLE BOWEL SYNDROME

This very common complaint is also called spastic colon or nervous bowel. It is characterized by colicky pain that usually occurs in the lower abdomen, a tendency to alternate between diarrhea and constipation, distension of the abdomen, wind, and sometimes heartburn. It may come and go over a very long period of time and is often aggravated by stress and tension.

Cause

There are conflicting theories about the origins of this problem, but it appears to be caused primarily by a lack of fiber – roughage – in the diet. By the time the nutrients have been absorbed from food, the remnants that reach the colon (large intestine) have insufficient bulk to enable them to be moved toward the rectum. Instead of the colon having to make small muscular contractions to squeeze a large bulk along its length, it has to make very tight contractions to propel a small bulk. This leads to muscle spasms and so causes pain. Stress amplifies the spasms and aggravates the pain. In fact, stress may be the factor that causes the activity in the colon to cross the pain and discomfort threshold in the first place.

The lack of bulk also produces either diarrhea or small, hard stools.

Treatment

From what has been said, it is clear that herbs to help stress and reduce muscular spasms, in addition to a change in diet and a more relaxed approach to life, are the basis of treatment. Relaxation exercises, yoga, and meditation have a lot to offer here. A re-evaluation of relationships, work, and life purpose often provides insights that, if acted upon, will remove the health problem.

Diet

Sometimes the simple addition of more roughage to the diet alleviates the problem, but may aggravate it if too much bran, or its equivalent, is added too quickly. An increase in fiber is best achieved through eating plenty of green vegetables, salads, fruits, and whole-grain bread. It may be appropriate to add bran to breakfast cereal or to eat it as bran cookies. Although it is dry, tasteless, and boring, bran can be made palatable by mixing it with other foods. Three tablespoons daily is enough.

Herbal remedies

Nature provides us with remedies that relax the digestive tract and ease the digestive process, in addition to providing relaxing nervines for the nervous system itself.

CHAMOMILE: This relaxing remedy gently eases the tensions in the digestive tract that cause the gripping pain.

FENNEL: A carminative that settles gripping colic and wind through the action of its oils.

HOPS: A moderately strong nervine relaxant. Also a sedative, as well as having a direct antispasmodic action.

PEPPERMINT: Apart from its wealth of other uses, the oil of peppermint is almost specific for calming digestive upsets such as irritable bowel syndrome.

WILD YAM: This remedy eases spasm and inflammation in the whole of the digestive tract.

The more specifically relaxing remedies should also be considered. These include valerian, scullcap, and many other remedies discussed elsewhere.

COLITIS

A number of difficult problems of the colon are intimately affected by tension and anxiety. These include ulcerative colitis and a less common problem called Crohn's disease. The symptoms are attacks of diarrhea that contains blood and mucus, and associated pain. Attacks are often precipitated or made worse by stress.

Cause

A lot of research has gone into how psychological factors contribute to ulcerative colitis. There appears to be not only a specific type of psychological stress that worsens the condition, but also a pattern of psychological characteristics that act as precursors.

Researchers have claimed that a high proportion of colitis sufferers tend to be obsessed with someone or something, are easily hurt, and find it difficult to express anger. While being outwardly energetic, ambitious, and efficient, they often feel inwardly insecure and inferior. They may be excessively dependent on a key person, with whom they often have an ambivalent relationship. Frequently this key person is the mother, who tends to control and dominate. On the whole, the families of sufferers tend to be restricted in their interactions and to show a false solidarity.

Certain kinds of life events seem more likely than others to trigger an attack. These are:

1. A real, threatened, or fantasized interruption of a key relationship. This could be the loss, or imagined loss, of someone close, such as a husband going to work temporarily in Alaska, or the fear of such a move.

2. An expectation of personal performance that the person feels unable to fulfill. This can take many forms, such as examinations, career goals, or relationships.

3. Disapproval from a parent figure – not only real parents, but anyone put into a position of respected authority.

Particularly important as triggers are situations where the person feels hostility and rage while also feeling helpless.

Treatment

Treatment of colitis conditions should not be undertaken by unskilled people. Colitis is a clear example of the way in which specific psychological patterns can contribute to specific physical problems. In addition to medical therapy, the use of counseling can provide insight into these nonphysical components, speed recovery, and open up the possibility of avoiding recurrence. It is especially helpful where the person feels unable to cope with his or her life the way it is.

The aim of psychotherapy should be to help the person become less vulnerable to the stresses of life. In addition, psychotherapy should help develop new ways to deal with the parent-figure. The themes of dependence and helplessness are ripe for such attention, and psychotherapy can do much to facilitate change and psychological healing. Another area for exploration is the way in which symptoms may be used as substitutes for more efficient ways of dealing with relationship problems. Illness is a good way to gain sympathy and power over the people we are close to, especially when the illness is all too real.

Herbal remedies have much to offer in the easing of colitis symptoms. If these remedies are used within the context of psychotherapy, then there is much hope of relief from this distressing and intransigent problem.

HEADACHES

Headaches must be our most common complaint. Turn on the television at any time and you'll see head pain depicted in advertisements for aspirin or its substitutes. Unfortunately, these drugs offer no lasting relief for chronic pain. If the roots of the headache are sought out and dealt with, the pain will go and not return.

Broadly speaking there are two types of headache: the muscular tension sort and the vascular or migraine sort. Both are aggravated or triggered by stress.

TENSION HEADACHES

Tension headaches are not only due to emotional tension. Tight muscles can also result from poor posture, from working in awkward positions, and from a too sudden strain. Stress, however, is the most common catalyst for transforming painless muscle tension into a headache.

Cause

As we have seen, stress is often emotional, but it can also be environmental. We might be irritated by the boss or by a pneumatic drill outside the window. Whatever the stimulus, the reaction is the same. Our muscles tense to prepare for fight or flight, to get away from the "threat." Since we usually don't take any action, tension builds up until the muscles become sore and cause pain.

Even though we are all under the stresses of our competitive society, not everyone suffers from chronic headaches. Why do some people collapse under the same pressures that others seem to thrive on? Each person has a different stress threshold, which allows one person to cope easily with major life events, while another suffers fits of anxiety in the face of a minor crisis. The anxious person is more prone to headaches.

Treatment

There are a number of better ways to approach headaches than simply taking aspirin. We will discuss a range of herbal remedies later, but just as important are attempts to ease the tension that is the root of the pain. This tension may be physical or psychological. Relaxation exercises were covered earlier in the book. Find one that suits you and use it regularly.

If the problem is in muscle tension, work with your body. It is possible that your posture, or the position you work in, is the culprit. A common cause of headaches in office workers is cupping the telephone between the shoulder and chin while writing. If you use the telephone a lot, this position will cause the muscles in your shoulder, neck, and head to contract and go into spasm. Soon they'll become painful and produce a headache even though you may otherwise be feeling calm and relaxed.

A simple exercise will help keep the neck and shoulders relaxed and poised. Whenever you feel tension around your head, sit back for a moment and do a few slow head rolls. Bring your chin down to your chest, slowly circle your head to the left, drop it back, then bring it to the right and back to your chest. It is best to do five rolls in one direction and then five in the other. These head rolls stretch the muscles that tend to get tense under pressure. This will help relieve any muscle spasms and so any consequent pain.

Herbal remedies

The advice given here for the easing of tension is generally useful for headaches. However, some herbs can produce headaches in sensitive people. The relaxing herb valerian has been known to do this. Ginseng (Panax ginseng, the Asiatic or American varieties) may cause headaches if used over too long a period, or at too high a dose.

Because this type of headache can be caused by a wide range of factors, there is a similarly wide range of remedies that have a reputation for easing head pain. It is best to study the additional virtues of the plants and choose those most appropriate in the broader context. A partial list includes:

Balm	Peppermint
Cayenne	Rosemary
Chamomile	Rue
Elder flower	Scullcap
Jamaica dogwood	Thyme
Lady's slipper	Valerian
Lavender	Wood betony
Marjoram	Wormwood

MIGRAINE

Most of the headaches that people describe as migraines are simply severe head pain. These can be bad enough, but migraines are in fact a specific type of headache that results from the constriction and dilation of blood vessels in the membranes that cover the brain. The process seems to be that a blood vessel first constricts but is then forced by the blood flow to dilate again. This dilation irritates the walls of the vessel, causing them to become inflamed and painful, and as the blood passes through the vessel, it produces a characteristic throbbing pain.

A migraine attack may start with visual phenomena that can look like flares around objects, or flashes of zig-zag patterns. The flare, or aura, seems to arise when a blood vessel constricts and causes a loss of blood to the brain. The pain that follows is severe and is often accompanied by nausea and vomiting, as well as a great sensitivity to light.

Cause

There appear to be a number of different causes for this traumatic problem. The roots of the migraine may, for example, originate in a spinal problem that could possibly be corrected by an osteopath or chiropractor. However, the most frequent triggers appear to be food, stress, and a change in hormone levels in women.

Treatment

For people whose migraines are triggered by stress, the various approaches to stress reduction suggested elsewhere in this book should be tried. Relaxation, meditation, and gently soothing exercise can provide much relief. It is well worth taking a close look at environmental conditions, such as working under fluorescent lighting or watching a computer screen all day. The physical environment and the quality of emotional relationships all play a large role in the generation of excess stress.

If there is any suspicion of back, neck, or cranial problems, it is worth consulting a good osteopath or chiropractor. Taking care of structural problems can often clear the migraines.

It is well established that foods containing tyramine, nitrite, monosodium glutamate, or alcohol are all capable of triggering migraines in sensitive people. Many books have been written about the dietary approach to the alleviation of migraine, so here I will just list the things to avoid. The most common triggers are:

Cheese
Chocolate
Eggs
Wheat and wheat products
Peanuts
Citrus fruits and tomatoes
Pork

To avoid these triggers, you will have to select foods that do not contain them in any form. In addition to these specific foods, it is worth avoiding tyramine-rich foods. These are:

Dairy products (especially cheese, yogurt, and sour cream)
Meat and fish (especially pickled herring, salted fish, sausage, and liver)
Some vegetables (broad beans, and sauerkraut)
Alcohol (especially beer, red wine, champagne, and sherry)

Migraines that occur because of hormone changes at the time of a period or menopause may seem intractable, but can be alleviated by using the correct herbal remedies. These remedies should be administered by a qualified medical herbalist, however, as is discussed below.

Herbal remedies

Many herbs are reputedly good for migraines. As has been pointed out, finding the correct one(s) depends upon being sure of the cause. One of Britain's best respected herbalists, Mrs. Gosling, has suggested the following easy-to-use mixture as a regular medicine:

"Motherwort, vervain, dandelion root, centaury, and wild carrot: each of these mixed together in equal parts and 25 g of this mixture simmered for fifteen minutes in 0.5 liters of water. A wineglass of this should be drunk three times a day."

Most of the remedies mentioned for tension headaches are of value, especially:

LAVENDER: Oil of lavender may be rubbed into the temples, or a couple of drops can be taken on a sugar cube. The flowers can be infused to make a tea.

FEVERFEW: This invaluable herb, while not quite the wonder remedy the media has led us to believe, will, with regular use—either fresh, as a tablet, or as tea—often clear migraines, given a month or so of treatment. If you have migraine, plant feverfew in your garden! It is best to use this herb fresh if at all possible.

HEART DISEASE

The blood that supplies oxygen and food to the heart moves through the coronary arteries that encircle the heart. If these arteries are narrowed, the blood supply is restricted and may become insufficient. The narrowing is usually due to the deposition on the walls of the blood vessels of a fatty substance called atheroma. If the blood supply is inadequate when an extra load is put on the heart—for example, during exercise or in cold weather—an angina attack may result. This involves a gripping pain across the chest and sometimes into the neck and jaw or down one or both arms. When the extra demand on the heart subsides, the pain passes.

Anxiety, fear, and stress may bring on such attacks, as there is an increase in adrenalin and noradrenaline release at such times. These hormones increase the work of the heart, making it beat faster. The pain experienced is itself a stress; sufferers become afraid of having an attack and the heightened anxiety makes one more likely.

A heart attack occurs when the blood supply to the heart muscle is abruptly stopped. This is often due to clotting in a coronary blood vessel. As we will see, stress can be a contributing factor here too. The details of this relationship are not entirely clear, but may be due to the fact that stress increases the stickiness of blood and makes it more likely to clot.

Cause

The origins of heart disease are complex and confusing. Some of the factors involved are well known and can lead to clear guidelines for possible prevention, but simplistic statements about saturated fats or jogging can be misleading. The search for factors that contribute to the scourge of heart disease has highlighted diet, personality type, socioeconomic conditions, and life events.

Diet

Whole forests have been turned into pulp to provide paper for articles about cholesterol, polyunsaturated fats, and heart disease. Anyone trying to read them all, or even follow the broad arguments, will get very stressed from the lack of agreement on the subject!

From the wealth of research done, it has been shown that heart disease has definite links with too much fat in the diet, raised blood cholesterol, raised blood pressure, smoking, obesity, short stature, and underactivity. The precise role of these factors is unclear, but enough is known to formulate general guidelines about a possible preventive diet.

Something that is certain is the involvement of fats. While the so-called saturated fats may be the worst, it seems that it is an over-preponderance of all fat in the total diet that is at fault. The way in which stress interacts with fats is partly as follows: A stressful life-style leads to the sustained production of the hormones adrenalin and noradrenaline. Among other actions, they mobilize fatty acids from the body's fat store, which provide a rapid source of energy. However, in the absence of exercise to use this energy, it is thought that the fatty acids accumulate and interact with other fatty substances to form yet another fatty substance called atheroma, which is deposited in plaques on the walls of blood vessels. This deposition does the most damage in the blood vessels close to the heart and in the brain and kidneys, because it causes a narrowing of the vessels and so limits the amount of blood available to these organs.

In this book, we do not explore specific diets in much depth, but these ideas are basic to avoiding heart problems:

1. Keep animal fats and cholesterol-rich foods to a minimum. These include red meat, dairy products, and eggs.

2. Use an absolute minimum of salt. Ideally, don't add any to food, either in cooking or at the table.

3. DON'T SMOKE!

4. Avoid excessive use of alcohol.

5. Generally avoid becoming overweight.

6. Avoid refined foods, such as white sugar and white bread; also avoid artificial additives of any kind.

Personality

An association between a particular type of personality and heart disease has been suggested for many years. As early as 1959, researchers were able to show that there was a difference in the risk of developing heart disease between people with two types of behavior, called type A and type B. We discussed these behavior types briefly in Chapter 2, but it might be useful to look at them a little closer.

Type A behavior is characterized by a chronic sense of time-urgency, aggressiveness (which may be repressed), and striving for achievement. Type A people often drive themselves to meet deadlines, many of which are self-imposed. They have feelings of being under pressure, both of time and responsibility, and often do two or three things at once. They are likely to react with hostility to anything that seems to get in their way and are temperamentally incapable of letting up. They are liable to think of themselves as indispensable. All of these factors add up to a state of constant stress!

Type B behavior is characterized by the opposite traits. Type B people are less preoccupied with achievement, less rushed, and generally more easygoing. They don't allow their lives to be governed by a sense of deadlines. They are less prone to anger and do not feel constantly impatient, rushed, and under pressure. They are also better at separating work from play, and they know how to relax.

Studies done over a period of eighteen months to two years with a group of type A and type B people showed that type A people had a 31 percent increased risk of developing heart disease.

Physical differences have been identified in people who exhibit one or the other of these two types of behavior. For example, there appear to be more plaque deposits in the coronary arteries of people who fit into the type A category. Type A behavior also has a close association with other medical risk factors, such as smoking, shortened blood-clotting time, higher-than-normal blood fat levels, and increased daily secretion of adrenalin, which in turn increases the oxygen requirement of the heart muscles and releases fatty acids from the body fat.

There is much debate about the methods used to assess type A behavior, the details of which do not concern us here. The important thing is the association of types of behavior with disease development. However, we need to bear in mind that there are not two types of people! Each person is an individual, and while it may sometimes be useful to sort people into artificial categories, these categories do not identify them.

Socioeconomic factors

A number of social and economic factors have been associated with an increased risk of heart disease; however, the findings tend to vary according to the society being studied. Some studies emphasize high risk in upper socioeconomic groups, while others emphasize the opposite. Some evidence suggests that class variation disappears when the degree of physical activity is taken into account.

High-risk socioeconomic factors appear to be:

1. Social mobility, which involves change of environment, such as moving to a new house or changing jobs.

2. Social incongruity, which is an inconsistency in people's status relevant to their life situation.

The relatively low occurrence of heart disease in women appears to be due to psychosocial rather than biological factors. Men are more likely to have an exaggerated striving for dominance and to use work as a major outlet for aggression, and so are more exposed to particular stresses and conflict and are more conditioned than women to "controlling" emotions when dealing with this conflict.

Such patterns seem to explain the difference between the incidence of heart disease in Western societies and in the Third World. Work pressures have hitherto been less intense in Third World countries, with family and social stability supporting and cushioning people from the frustrations that characterize the pattern in the West.

Many ideas have been put forward to try and explain Western civilization's predisposition to heart disease. For example:

1. It occurs through the need for self-discipline, intellectual control, and distant goals rather than basic drives and their more immediate gratification.

2. The modern environment encourages high-risk, type A behavior by rewarding haste, aggressive competition, and a constant excessive preoccupation with the demands of work schedules.

Life events

Particularly stressful times in a person's life act as possible danger points in stress-related problems such as heart disease. When these stressful times are identified, it is possible to take them into account and plan ahead. This makes it possible to manage and lessen the impact of these stresses on health and well-being. As we have discussed, there are well-known points of increased stress, called life events, in everyone's life. These are especially relevant in the development of conditions such as angina and heart disease, and it is worth becoming familiar with them and learning how to prepare for them.

Treatment

The treatment of heart disease must be undertaken by a skilled practitioner. For the best possible results, it is essential, however, that sufferers be involved in their own treatment. This might sound like a truism, but unfortunately we have become isolated from our own healing processes by the very expertise of medical doctors and even of alternative practitioners such as herbalists.

Patient involvement is especially important when the emotional aspects of the disease are considered. It comes as no surprise that a great reduction in the chances of repeat attacks or the development of complications is achieved with the successful management of psychological and social problems. Methods of dealing with anxiety and tension must be found that will suit the person involved. For some people, self-help techniques like relaxation exercises are not enough, and they may need help with anxiety and tension that has its roots in self-image, belief systems, relationships, work goals, environment, and so on. Treatment should be based on a broad reappraisal of life-style and life goals, not simply on medical approaches to the illness. Diet, exercise, relaxation, meditation, and other stress-reduction techniques are all potentially appropriate, and are described throughout the book.

Herbal remedies

Herbal remedies have a lot to offer in the treatment, prevention, and alleviation of heart problems. *It must be emphasized, however, that any herbal treatment of the heart must be undertaken under the supervision of a well-trained medical herbalist,* especially if the heart is already being treated with drugs.

A number of remedies have a direct action on the heart itself. These include:

Broom
Hawthorn berries
Lily of the valley
Lime blossom
Mistletoe

You will notice that I haven't included the well-known heart herb foxglove. In modern medical herbalism, this is considered poisonous and is only used under specific circumstances. It should never be used in the home.

In addition to the herbs with specific heart actions, a whole range of herbs can be used to aid and support the heart by generally helping the body. These herbs are discussed in other sections.

There is much that can be done with herbs to help the stress that accompanies and contributes to heart problems. These are all considered in much more depth in other parts of the book, but it is worth pointing out one that has particular relevance when the heart is involved:

MOTHERWORT: Its Latin name (Leonurus cardiaca) shows how motherwort's reputation for aiding the heart has been recognized by botanists (cardiac means "related to the heart"). It can be used for palpitations.

Other relaxing plants that may prove useful include the following (remember, though, that different remedies may suit some people more than others):

Balm
St. John's wort
Scullcap

HYPERACTIVITY IN CHILDREN

Hyperactivity is a growing area of concern, because its causes seem so all-pervasive. It is clear that artificial food additives have a lot to answer for here. It appears that young, developing nervous systems are particularly prone to the damage or irritation that many food additives can cause. The effect is one of excessive activity with only a few hours sleep each night, and because of the overactivity, the sufferers are more prone to accidents. There is some association with eczema and asthma, both of which are aggravated by overactivity. There may also be difficulties with speech, balance, and learning, even if the child has a high IQ.

Anyone with a child who is suspected of having this problem will be under extreme stress themselves. So there are two things to look at: ways to help the child, and ways to help the parents.

Excellent support groups have been formed that are sources

of useful information about this problem. Look in your Yellow Pages for local groups or contact The Feingold Association, 56 Winston Drive, Smithtown, NY 11787 (516 543-4658). Send a stamped, self-addressed envelope for their reply.

Treatment

One treatment that can be quite effective is based on a diet developed by Dr. Feingold. It requires cutting out of the diet all foods and drinks containing synthetic additives of any kind, as well as certain natural chemicals. For more specific details contact The Feingold Association at the address given above. A combination of this diet and good herbal treatment for any physical symptoms the child has developed should help clear the problem.

Herbal remedies

Herbal relaxants that may help hyperactive children include the following, which are best used as an infusion added to a bath (see Chapter 9, "How to Prepare Herbal Remedies," for more information):

RED CLOVER: A gentle relaxing remedy that helps the liver and also clears the skin of minor eruptions.

LIME BLOSSOM: This is stronger, though still a mild, relaxing herb.

CHAMOMILE: An all-round relaxing plant that is especially good for children.

As I've said, it is the parents, more than the child, who often need herbs for stress and tension. Any parent supporting a hyperactive child would benefit from the advice given in chapter two on how to deal with long-term stress.

INSOMNIA

Good sleep is fundamental to good health, and lack of sleep will hurt, either immediately or eventually. On a day-to-day basis, pain, stress, and anxiety may all be disruptive to a good night's sleep, leaving you fatigued the next day. This fatigue reduces the body's ability to cope with stress and discomfort, so that you become even more uncomfortable and probably more anxious. This makes it more likely that the following night's sleep will be upset. And so you enter into a vicious cycle of stress/insomnia/fatigue/increased stress/more insomnia/greater fatigue....

Lack of sleep may be voluntary; you may stay up to watch a late show on television or to go to a party, for example. Getting less sleep than optimum for extended periods may also be by choice. The body may appear to adapt to operating while tired, but continued lack of sleep will tell in the long run via serious disease or disorder, increased vulnerability to stress symptoms, and faster aging.

Treatment

Never try to fall asleep. Sleep isn't "done," it just happens when your mind and body are ready. The best you can do is clear away the things that may be keeping you awake, such as unconscious muscle tension. If you're both mentally and physically restless and can't get comfortable, don't fight it: get up and do something – anything – for a short while, even though you're not really interested. Force yourself. You'll soon feel tired enough to try falling asleep again.

Obviously, you should make sure that your bed is as comfortable as possible. Use pillows in such a way that your neck and head are in line with your spine, with no awkward twists or bends. And be sure your bedding is firm enough to support your body evenly, especially along the spine, without sagging.

Sometimes dietary changes can help. For example, a very light snack an hour before going to bed may help some people. A sandwich made with lettuce seems particularly helpful, perhaps because commercial lettuce is the cultivated cousin of the wild species. Other than taking this light snack (if it helps), do not eat for at least three to four hours before going to bed. Eating not only stimulates your metabolism just when it should be slowing down, but eating at bedtime is also a major factor in the gain of excess weight. It may be all right to drink something, but definitely stay away from caffeine drinks, such as tea, coffee, hot chocolate, and colas.

The natural amino acid L-tryptophan taken regularly for about a month will usually help the sleep process. This amino acid is a natural precursor to a sleep-inducing chemical found in the brain. Another supplement that can help is dolomite tablets.

Relaxation exercises

If you wake up in the middle of the night and can't fall back to sleep within ten to fifteen minutes, then try some simple relaxation exercises. The relaxation exercises discussed elsewhere in the book will help you ease into sleep. Give them a try. For some people, the relaxation and sleep-aiding cassettes that are now available have proven quite useful.

If you use the exercises described in this book to help with insomnia, continue until you either fall asleep or complete the entire exercise. Do the exercises lying on your back, even though you may be used to falling asleep on your side. Either you'll fall asleep on your back, which is good for you, or you'll turn onto your side as you lose focus and begin to drift off.

If you complete the routine and yet are still mentally awake, don't be concerned that you are not actually asleep, because by this time your body is deeply relaxed. You are getting excellent physical rest anyway, and it's usually true that if you're really relaxed but not asleep, your brain doesn't really need sleep at this time. In this situation, enjoy yourself: dream, fantasize, speculate, ponder decisions that need making, consider problems that need solving, and so forth. Your body is relaxed, so don't be afraid to let your mind be active. Many people find this physically calm, mentally clear state very attractive and productive. If you think of something you want to write down, get up and do so. You won't spoil any magical physical state. In fact, upon returning to bed you may fall asleep more readily than ever.

Usually, however, you will fall asleep long before completing the relaxation exercise. In fact, you may wake up the next morning and not remember getting any further than your legs! But don't be concerned with when and if you actually fall asleep. Remember, you can't control that, anyway. And any attention you give to such thoughts as "Am I asleep yet?" doesn't help you to fall asleep any sooner. In fact, your worry may do just the opposite and make you stay awake longer. Instead of focusing on whether you're asleep yet, or on any discomfort you feel, or on the house sounds you can hear, focus on breathing and muscle awareness each night until you are either asleep or so deeply relaxed physically that it doesn't matter.

Herbal remedies

Nature is rich in plant remedies that help sooth the sometimes stormy route to sleep. If the mind won't stop racing or the body is agitated, or sleep escapes you for no good reason at all, herbs can be a real help.

The strong and potentially dangerous narcotic plants are, of course, illegal and won't be discussed here. All the plants I will mention are safe and nonaddictive. They can be used in a number of ways. Specific details are discussed in the chapter on preparation, but to aid sleep, herbal remedies are most effective taken as teas or used as additives in baths. Bath additives made with relaxing plants that have a pleasant aroma work best. The combination of a relaxing nervine herb such as a few drops of lavender oil added to a bath, followed by a cup of sleep-inducing valerian tea is both pleasant and effective.

All the relaxing remedies discussed elsewhere in the book may be sufficient to help soothe the body and mind enough for sleep to come. Herbs such as scullcap, lavender, and motherwort, while not primarily for insomnia, may have the desired effect. Here I will list the plants with a reputation for inducing sleep.

HOPS: This traditional remedy is still used in the form of hop pillows to help with sleep; but more often it is taken as a tea.

JAMAICA DOGWOOD: A good relaxing remedy that also has mild pain-relieving properties.

LIME BLOSSOM: This gentle relaxing remedy is safe for children. It makes a good herb pillow and is especially good for its beneficial effects on the circulation.

PASSIONFLOWER: One of the best sleep-producing plants, passionflower is used in most proprietary mixtures. The right dosage varies from person to person, so experiment, building up the strength over a few nights.

VALERIAN: Use this good relaxing nervine during the day for anxiety and tension, and at night if your sleep is disturbed by anxious thoughts. This herb does not suit everyone, however, so if you get headaches or do not feel at all better, do not continue with it. Try another remedy.

WILD LETTUCE: For some people, this remedy can be a

strong sedative; unfortunately, for others, it may not always work.

With the wide range of plants that can help and the different ways to use them, we would need a separate book to explore all the combinations of herbs that might be used for sleep. So I'll just mention a particular favorite of mine. This is a mixture of equal parts of scullcap, valerian, and passionflower, which makes an effective sleep potion. It can be made by mixing equal parts of either the dried herbs or their tinctures. If using the dried herbs, then let an ounce of the herb mixture infuse in a pint of boiling water for ten minutes. If insomnia is a major problem, then take one wineglassful (4 fluid ounces) of this tea after each meal and two before going to bed.

PAIN

It may come as a surprise, but pain is not an illness. It is a subjective sensation, and has been described as an emotion. It usually accompanies some physical ill and often acts as an early warning sign. As such, pain plays a valuable role in health – not that it should be welcomed, but rather listened to. This is the most worrying aspect of the enormous consumption of painkillers today. Not only physical but also emotional pain is being masked and suppressed when it should be listened to.

The experience of pain is often amplified or reduced by our previous experiences of pain and its relief, as well as by our ability (or inability) to cope with it. Physical pain may become much worse when we are under any form of stress. A good example is a backache that gets much worse when we find out we are overdrawn at the bank. Thus, different people have different pain thresholds and it is very difficult to comprehend another's experience of pain.

Pain can cause anxiety and depression, especially when associated with chronic illness.

Treatment

From this brief discussion, it is clear that pain as such is not what we should focus on. Primarily, we should attend to the roots of the pain, and should use painkillers only within the broader treatment of the pain's cause.

Appropriate treatment of any pain related to structural problems might rest in the hands of a chiropractor or osteopath. Acupuncture also has a lot to offer, and it is becoming increasingly clear that many headaches have their origin in jaw problems that good dentists may be able to help with.

Herbal remedies

As I've said, herbs are the basis of most of the pharmaceutical drugs used today. All the morphine- and cocaine-type painkillers and anesthetics come originally from plants. None of the stronger painkillers are freely available, for obviously they must only be used under qualified observation. In the current state of medical monopoly, this prevents qualified medical herbalists from using such herbs – an unfortunate state of affairs!

Some gentle herbs that can relieve pain are more readily available, but once again I want to emphasize that the cause of the pain must be sought. Safe herbs worth considering include the following:

ST. JOHN'S WORT: Especially valuable for long-standing neuralgic pain. It is used internally or as an external application for at least three weeks.

JAMAICA DOGWOOD: This herb is also a mild sedative.

VALERIAN: Aids in anxiety reactions that might accompany pain.

YELLOW JASMINE: This is a much stronger pain reliever that should be used only under skilled herbal advice.

WILD LETTUCE: A good relaxing pain reliever. The wild variety is now rather rare.

The plants listed above are for pain in general, but that is not very common! If pain is due to muscle spasms, then try antispasmodic herbs; if due to external problems, use vulnerary ones. A complete list of the herbs to consider would be almost endless, but bear in mind that anxiety will aggravate and be aggravated by pain.

RHEUMATOID ARTHRITIS

Rheumatoid arthritis is characterized by swelling, pain, and stiffness of the joints. It is quite different in origin to the more common osteoarthritis. This increasingly prevalent disease is undoubtedly aggravated by stress of any kind. As already pointed out, it is one of the so-called autoimmune conditions, all of which are made worse by anxiety and tension.

In rheumatoid arthritis there is a proliferation of inflammatory tissue in the membranes that line some of the body's joints. The specific cause is unknown but is directly related to the body's immune system, which for some reason, turns against the protein in the body's own joint linings. This causes the painful inflammation and eventually destruction of tissue.

Treatment

Among the factors that disturb the immune system in predisposed people is the impact of stress, so any effective treatment of this difficult illness must include a stress management program that is relevant to the person involved. An easing of tension and anxiety must be a priority.

Diet also plays a role in the aggravation and possibly even the origin of rheumatoid arthritis. The possible ramifications of dietary adjustment are complex, so advice should be sought from a skilled practitioner. Basically, emphasis is on low acid and no dairy products, with an avoidance of all artificial additives. The role of diet in the treatment of rheumatoid arthritis is a contentious area. A list of books on the subject of dietary disease control is included in the bibliography.

Herbal remedies

Herbal medicine has a lot to offer, but because rheumatoid arthritis is a deep-seated problem based in the immune system, it is impossible to talk of specific remedies. A good herbalist will be of much help. The following plants have a role in any broad treatment regimen, which must take into account the unique situation of the person involved. Remember that to truly help, the whole person must be treated, which means that more than just the joint condition may need to be taken into account.

BLACK COHOSH: This useful cleansing and relaxing herb aids in reducing inflammation.

BOGBEAN: One of the best all-round remedies for arthritic conditions. Also acts on the liver, and aids digestion and general body cleansing.

CELERY SEED: This is an excellent remedy with a specific affinity for the skeleton and musculature. It is worth any one prone to arthritis making celery a major part of the diet.

MEADOWSWEET: Among the wealth of attributes of this useful, all-round remedy is its ability to reduce inflammation in the joints.

WILD YAM: This herb is the natural origin of synthetic steroids. It can aid in acutely inflamed arthritis, and is also used in digestive problems such as diverticulitis.

WILLOW BARK: A rich source of natural aspirin that does not have any of the potential problems of the synthetic drug. Can be used to ease pain in the joints.

SKIN DISEASE

The skin often acts as a form of body semaphore that allows the stress experienced elsewhere in the body or in the mind to express itself on the surface. It often is a cry for help or for attention to a problem whose existence we have tried to deny. It is this denial that makes it necessary for the problem to appear on the skin. This perception gives us a powerful way of approaching skin disease. Through counseling and supportive psychotherapy, much can be done to ease the impact of conditions such as psoriasis, and so reverse the momentum of the illness and speed its clearing.

Cause

The skin is affected by many different things, from simple infections to allergies to the more complex and obscure autoimmune problems. Most skin conditions are aggravated by anxiety and tension and some are actually brought on by stress itself. This is especially true of a form of eczema called atopic eczema, and of psoriasis. While psoriasis is not an emotionally based illness as many consider it to be, it often, of itself, acts as an emotional stress. In fact, the emotional stress caused by psoriasis is often one of the worst features of the condition.

Emotional factors and stress are important in the development, aggravation, and perpetuation of many skin diseases, and the stress and even misery caused by a skin disease may cause a vicious circle. An awareness by friends, relatives, and the general public that such conditions are not contagious and are not dirty, and that the disease is not the sufferer's fault and actually causes him or her great embarrassment, would help reduce the stress caused by skin disease and make the treatment a lot easier.

Treatment

All holistic approaches to medicine have a lot to offer in treating skin disease. Dietary approaches are especially indicated in skin problems, but this is an area that goes beyond the range of this book.

Herbal remedies

Used internally as systemic aids and externally as ointments and lotions, herbal remedies are particularly helpful. The list of possible remedies is endless, but here are some suggestions:

BURDOCK ROOT: A good general remedy for chronic skin problems. Also aids the digestion and assimilation of food because of the way it works on the liver. It is especially useful in psoriasis and rheumatism.

CHICKWEED: Used as a lotion or ointment, or in a bath, it reduces irritation, sometimes quite dramatically.

CLEAVERS: This common plant specifically works on the lymphatic system and so helps one of the body's own cleansing systems. It is useful for all skin problems.

FIGWORT: Widely used for skin problems. Acts as a general tonic.

GOLDEN SEAL: One of the herbs that comes close to being a "cure all"! Because of its broadly beneficial action on the body, it aids in most skin problems. It is a good lotion for eczema and skin infections like ringworm, especially when combined in equal parts with marigold or myrrh.

MARIGOLD: The flowers, used internally or externally, are especially useful in eczema. This is one of the best wound healers and is specific for fungal infections.

MYRRH: This "old-fashioned" remedy makes a good external wash for infections.

YELLOW DOCK: Good for chronic skin conditions. It is also a mild laxative.

This is only a small selection of the plant remedies available. In addition, the nervine relaxant herbs described elsewhere can be helpful. One that is worth a special mention here is:

RED CLOVER: This gentle skin remedy is specific in some types of childhood eczema. It also has a mild relaxing action and aids restful sleep, reducing itching and thereby causing less scratching.

STRESS PROBLEMS OF WOMEN

In Western society, all kinds of emotional and mental disorders are more common in women than in men. This bald fact opens up vast areas of psychological, sociological, physiological, and political exploration, most of which are inappropriate for discussion here. However, I'd like to point out that the atmosphere that presently pervades our society could easily be viewed as evidence of mental illness on the part of the patriarchy that runs it. The alienation and depersonalization of our cities, militarism, multinational corporate oppression, the nuclear threat, and an inequality of world resources that has lead to massive misery could all be seen as aspects of the prevalence of male mental disorders!

That aside, we will focus here on the "syndromes" common to women. Two main reasons have been suggested for the higher incidence of mental disorders in women than in men: genetic factors and the social pressures on women that result from upbringing and cultural expectations. It might seem a bit pretentious for a male herbalist to try and comprehend how herbs can help with "female" problems, but what I will focus on are those health problems that most commonly feed patterns of stress and anxiety, and the ways that herbs can ease them. The broader issues of relationships and cultural roles I will but hint at.

An herbal that is full of deep compassion and comprehension in this area is *Hygieia* by Jeannine Parvati. I strongly recommend its insights.

PREMENSTRUAL SYNDROME

Premenstrual syndrome (PMS) is a condition that was until recently denied official existence! It was put down to "hysterical female behavior" – of course, by male doctors. It can be described as a condition of physical, behavioral, and mood changes related to the menstrual cycle. The most common symptoms, including irritability, depression, breast tenderness, and a "bloated" sensation, are found in many cultures and ethnic groups. There is an increased rate of appeals to suicide prevention centers and women are more likely to enter hospitals as psychiatric emergencies during their premenstrual period. Pre-existing disorders such as migraine or skin problems are likely to be exacerbated, and life generally becomes more of a strain, the degree of pressure varying from one woman to another.

Cause

Little clarity has come from physiological research into the causes of this problem. Localized water retention in various parts of the body has been implicated as a possible cause of the tension, as have hormonal changes. Cyclical changes in certain brain chemicals have also been suggested.

There is no doubt that marked body changes do occur, but all such physiological work ignores, to its loss, the powerful involvement of the mind and emotions in PMS and in menstruation in general. It has been suggested that premenstrual and menstrual problems are a conditioned pattern of response to hormonal changes that result from the woman's experience of her mother's attitudes and approaches to periods. If these attitudes were not open and healthy, then as a child, the woman may have developed resistance and psychological blockage around the whole subject. As she grew and matured, this would surface as premenstrual tension.

There are many other such theories, the point being that this disruptive and unpleasant problem probably has a range of causative factors feeding it. There is no one "thing" to blame.

Treatment

The use of vitamin B_{12} has been advocated in the treatment of PMS and is often suggested by doctors; however, evidence of its efficacy is equivocal.

Both supportive and insight psychotherapy have a valuable role to play, as do relaxation and possibly meditation techniques, all of which are discussed elsewhere in the book.

Herbal remedies

Herbal remedies such as the following can prove extremely successful in the short-term relief and long-term improvement of PMS. These remedies are best used when the problem is active, just before menstruation starts.

SCULLCAP: This valuable remedy can be considered a specific for the relief of the emotional and mental symptoms of PMS. It may be combined with other effective tension-relieving remedies, including the following:

CRAMP BARK: A generally mild relaxing herb that is very effective in easing the cramps that may be associated with PMS.

MOTHERWORT: This perennial herb may be useful in tension-relieving combinations because of its relaxing properties plus its safe action in reducing stress-related palpitations.

PASQUE FLOWER: A valuable relaxing plant that helps when tearful emotion gets out of hand. Remember, though, that tears are good for you!

VALERIAN: This is widely used with benefit in PMS, especially where there is cramping or overagitation.

Choice of specific remedies will obviously depend upon prior knowledge of what works best for you, but should also take into account the degree of associated symptoms, such as cramping and water retention. This might make choosing a remedy sound a bit complex, but it is in fact quite straightforward.

In the context of a balanced herbal approach to the person's whole being, long-term treatment is best based on the use of:

CHASTEBERRY: This works over a period of time to balance hormone levels without interfering with any of the body's necessary work.

Herbs that remove water from the body – diuretics – are sometimes suggested for the relief of PMS. The value of diuretics is debatable, however, as water retention may be secondary to emotional tension rather than the other way around. Thus scullcap may relieve the water retention while diuretics may not ease the tension. If diuretics are suggested, then consider:

Dandelion leaf
Bearberry
Yarrow

These are only suggestions. Each woman is unique and occasionally remedies reputed to have specific actions do not do a thing.

PSYCHOLOGICAL PROBLEMS OF PREGNANCY

Pregnancy, particularly the first one, is a psychological watershed. The transition to motherhood is a creative process in which fundamental changes in the concept of self and of role are negotiated against a background of resolved and still unsettled developmental "crises." The psychological and physical demands of the infant are an essential ingredient in this process of maturation, which begins, however, long before the baby is born. For the pregnant woman, becoming a mother means becoming a different sort of child of her own parents, a different sort of sexual partner, and indeed a different sort of mother if there are already children in the family. Temporary or permanent changes of career and of social role can be a direct consequence of pregnancy and are sometimes a source of major difficulty.

Treatment

For women with no previous history of mental ill health, the minor psychological problems that do arise during pregnancy can be dealt with by increased support from midwives, doctors, and herbalists, but most especially from the family. There is a need for clear and informed reassurance, prenatal classes, and sharing with other mothers.

Anticipating the impact that a life event such as pregnancy can have on the mind and emotions reduces the chances of a woman developing severe mental problems. Of course, this is as it should be, highlighting the inherent health and wholeness of this most holistic of "life events."

Ten to 35 percent of pregnant women take some form of tranquilizer or sleeping pill. All of the drugs that can cross the blood-brain barrier can also cross into the placenta. Higher blood levels of the drug then develop in the fetus than in the mother, and this leads to sedation of the baby. The inappropriateness and danger of this should be quite clear. The use of supportive counseling, marriage therapy, and herbal nervines is obviously preferable.

Problems associated with miscarriage, stillbirth, or abortion greatly benefit from the help of an experienced and skilled counselor.

All the herbs that ease anxiety and tension are usually quite safe for use during pregnancy, but if they are needed often, it is best to consult a qualified practitioner.

POSTNATAL DEPRESSION

About 10 percent of women develop depression after childbirth. Onset is usually within the first month. Investigations to find metabolic causes are inconclusive, but often point to psychological and social factors, such as marital disharmony, poor housing, and financial problems. In one research study, postnatal depression was found more frequently in women who had had doubts about continuing their pregnancies and in those who had difficulties in relationships with their own parents.

Any difficulties in adjusting to being a mother are likely to be exacerbated by such symptoms of depression as increased irritability, lowered self-esteem, guilt, and inability to cope. Moreover, depression may have repercussions on the child. What should be a time of joy and coming together thus becomes one of stress and tension. Some mothers express inner conflicts by an inability to allow the child a separate existence, and they scrutinize the baby's every movement. Although they complain about exhaustion and misery, they are often resistant to counseling and support.

Treatment

Postnatal depression usually passes within a few months and its passage can be considerably speeded by simple supportive measures, including reduction of any sense or experience of isolation, identification of sources of stress, and then their avoidance or removal. Sharing of feeding responsibilities often helps both parents at this time of profound reorientation.

Apart from such support, advice to ensure adequate diet and appropriate herbal medication will ease matters. The advice of a qualified herbalist must be sought for this problem. Herbs other than nervines and antidepressants may be recommended, as there is a need to aid the body in its task of recuperation and breast-feeding.

MENOPAUSE

Menopause is one of the biggest transitions a human being can go through. Much has been written about its multiple problems; however, it can also be a time of new freedom. The ties of a lifetime and the roles with which society has bound a woman can at last be loosened.

The undoubted physical problems of the hormonal transformation can be eased and in some cases removed altogether. Whether the hormonal changes are what cause the rather too common mental and emotional problems is unclear, since this is often a time of major life events, such as children leaving home, parents dying, and husband retiring.

Treatment

There can be no doubt that this time period has profound implications for the woman involved, who may view the major changes in her personal role as rendering her "useless." Counseling work based on an exploration of the opportunities that open up in the "change of life" can be valuable, especially if the woman can come to see this time as a new start, where she can create what she wants and not simply what her children and husband need, if these previously defined her activities. Menopause thus becomes a release rather than a reason for being rejected, no matter what she is changing from and moving to.

Herbal remedies

Herbal remedies can help with both the hormonal and the psychological problems. Herbs to consider include:

BLUE COHOSH: This is an American Indian plant that balances and normalizes the function of the whole of the female reproductive system.

CHASTEBERRY: A valuable remedy from the Eastern Mediterranean that balances hormonal traumas and has a profound action in lessening "hot flashes."

FALSE UNICORN ROOT: This root is similar in broad action to blue cohosh.

GOLDEN SEAL: An excellent remedy for all-round health, specifically for the toning of mucous membranes, such as those that line the uterus and vagina.

LADY'S MANTLE: Named from its leaf shape. Has similar properties to chasteberry, although not as strong.

LIFE ROOT: This perennial root is similar in broad action to blue cohosh.

A whole range of the herbal relaxing and antidepressant remedies may be indicated. The specifics will vary from woman to woman and so should ideally be prescribed by a good herbalist. Certain plants are worth emphasizing:

MOTHERWORT: This nervine can be most useful when hot flashes are compounded by palpitations. It is a safe, relaxing remedy.

PASQUE FLOWER: A relaxing herb that reduces the anxiety and occasional irrationality produced by menopausal changes.

ST. JOHN'S WORT: Apart from its wide range of uses for many other bodily systems, this wonderful remedy is almost specific for depression and tension associated with menopause.

SCULLCAP: This is a widely applicable relaxing remedy.

VALERIAN: This is a good herb to use when stronger sedating may be called for.

TEN

Antianxiety Drugs: How to Kick the Habit

The usual result of going to the doctor for help with problems of anxiety or depression is a prescription. It is unfortunate that traditional health services have become so pressured by the demands made on them that they should perhaps now be called "disease" services. While there is no doubt that doctors and nurses valiantly do their best to care for their patients, in the case of "nerve" conditions, it seems that the most expedient thing to do is throw vast amounts of drugs at the problem. As we have discussed throughout this book, such an approach is short-sighted and potentially dangerous.

For people with major psychological problems, there can be no doubt that drug therapy has much to offer. In the treatment of schizophrenia and psychosis in general, great advances have been made through the use of drugs. However, the use of drugs in the treatment of the so-called "neuroses" can mask the basic problems and, unfortunately, lead to the development of new ones. Anyone taking drugs for a psychological condition should know what they are being given and what side effects may occur, including withdrawal effects when the time comes to stop taking the drug.

This chapter will present a brief review of the drugs commonly prescribed for some psychological conditions and their possible side effects. The drugs reviewed are used for anxiety, tension, and their associated manifestations. No mention is made of antidepressant drugs or those used in the treatment of major psychological problems. This review is meant to be used as a reference only. The side effects mentioned are those that medical experience has shown can occur. This does not mean that they will necessarily occur in your case. Following the review, we will discuss some ways that herbs can help ease the withdrawal from certain kinds of drugs.

SEDATIVES AND HYPNOTICS

A broad approach to help alleviate insomnia and sleep disturbance was discussed in the previous chapter. This section deals with the possible impact of the various drugs that are commonly prescribed to "help" with this problem.

Sedatives and hypnotics are drugs that depress brain function. In small doses, they are used to calm and reduce tension, and are called sedatives. In larger doses, they are used to induce sleep, and are called hypnotics. All such drugs are potentially addictive and can quickly produce psychological dependence. This dependence is strengthened by the fact that when we stop taking these drugs, we often go through a period of restless sleep, the very condition the drugs were prescribed to relieve. In fact, as we discussed earlier, they are often unnecessary in the first place.

If taken regularly at a dosage level above that recommended, they cause intoxication. Elderly and debilitated people, or people with heart, kidney, or liver problems, may develop intoxication at "normal" dosage levels. The signs of intoxication include confusion, difficulty in speaking, unsteadiness, poor memory, faulty judgment, irritability, excessive emotion, hostility, suspiciousness, and even suicidal tendencies.

All drugs in this group can produce physical dependence and resultant withdrawal symptoms if they are suddenly stopped. These may include anxiety, trembling, weakness, dizziness, nausea, vomiting, convulsions, delirium, and – rarely – death. Compared with the number of people taking these drugs, the number who develop physical dependence is rare, but psychological dependence is very common. Tolerance to the drugs is also common and leads to less effect from the same dosage over time. This carries the danger that the dosage will be increased to obtain the same effect, raising the chances of addiction.

This category of drugs, and especially the barbiturates, can produce anxiety, irritability, and depression as side effects, and since the drugs have often been prescribed to ease these very symptoms, again there may be a temptation simply to raise the dosage. In some cases, the drugs actually make things worse, and there is some evidence that drug-induced sleep does not have the restorative functions of normal sleep.

One sign that the drugs may be causing possible problems is if, after using a drug to help sleep, the person awakes feeling less tense, only to become tired, irritable, and bad tempered later in the day. The drug may impair learned behaviors and the ability to concentrate.

Barbiturates

Barbiturates are among the oldest synthetic sedatives and have been in use for almost a hundred years. They are prescribed in the treatment of anxiety, tension, and restlessness, as well as for sleep problems. The barbiturates used to produce sleep have an effect that lasts for about eight hours, and all cause some degree of "hangover." They entail a high risk of psychological and physiological dependence. They have largely been replaced by the benzodiazepines, which are discussed later in this chapter in the "Minor Tranquilizer" section.

A large number of brands of barbiturates are available on prescription, including: phenobarbitone, Amytal, Amytal Sodium, Nembutal, and Seconal.

Nonbarbiturate Hypnotics

A diverse group of nonbarbiturate drugs can be used to induce sleep. Many, such as bromide and chloral hydrate (a Mickey Finn), are rarely used now. All the drugs in this group have the potential of producing tolerance and addiction, increase the effects of alcohol, interfere with the ability to concentrate and drive, and cause intoxication.

Brand names include Doriden, Noludar, and Placidyl.

Antihistamines

The antihistamines, which are usually used for the suppression of allergy reactions, produce drowsiness as a side effect. This is sometimes used to promote sleep.

MINOR TRANQUILIZERS

Another category of drugs is used primarily to treat anxiety and tension. By far the most important group here are the benzodiazepines, which are also prescribed for sleeping problems.

Benzodiazepines

The benzodiazepines are the most widely prescribed antianxiety drugs. They are used for anxiety, insomnia, muscular tension, and convulsions, and to ease withdrawal from other drugs.

A host of adverse effects can accompany their use. They can cause confusion and interfere with the ability to concentrate, to use machinery, or to drive safely. The most common effects are drowsiness and lethargy. They may also cause a fall in blood pressure and stimulate the appetite. Headaches may occur, as well as dizziness and nausea. Sometimes excitement results, so that instead of becoming calm, the person looks and acts as if drunk. These drugs increase the effects of alcohol and have been an agent in accidental or intentional overdose. It is now clear that they can produce a form of physical dependence, and withdrawal can be a problem unless approached the right way (this will be discussed in a moment).

The benzodiazepines include, among many others, the following brand names: Librium, Valium, Ativan, Dalmane, and Tranxene. Any of these will induce sleep at high dosages.

HERBAL MEDICINE AND BENZODIAZEPINE DEPENDENCE

The herbalist is not the practitioner best-suited to deal with the growing problem of drug abuse and dependency; however, plants have so much to offer in easing withdrawal from the benzodiazepines that it is worth exploring the undoubted value of herbs and counseling in this context. We will not concern ourselves here with the disturbing "street" use of these drugs, where dangerously high doses may be taken to produce euphoria and intoxication. Rather, we will address the needs of those who originally used one of the benzodiazepines for temporary relief from stress and anxiety, but who now find that the drug has itself become the problem.

It is unfortunately safe to assume that a very large number of people are long-term benzodiazepine users and so can be considered "dependent." Repeatedly prescribing these drugs has serious social consequences, the most important of which are the effects on the individual. Long-term users may experience what has been called "emotional anesthesia" and a marked lowering of scores in objective psychological tests. Although the original symptoms of most long-term users no longer exist, the repeat prescribing continues for reasons other than the original need, sometimes because it is simply too hard to stop taking the drug.

A dose in excess of 40 mg daily will, after three months, produce minor withdrawal symptoms if stopped, and some sensitive people will experience these symptoms with smaller doses over a shorter period. People who have been taking these drugs for months or years may have increased the dosage level to achieve symptom relief, and when it is abruptly discontinued, more serious withdrawal symptoms may occur. These may range from anxiety and depression, through severe emotional and perceptual changes to (rarely) convulsions. The anxiety will be similar to that for which the drug was prescribed in the first place and so prompt the recommencement of treatment. The other symptoms can be rather frightening and can include such things as insomnia, nausea, malaise, and depersonalization, as well as perceptual changes such as shimmering lights, loud noises, unsteadiness, and a sensation of motion.

The incidence and impact of such distressing withdrawal symptoms can be greatly alleviated by a step-by-step reduction in dosage, accompanied by the appropriate herbal medication, which acts as a bridge. While you can carry out a withdrawal plan on your own, it is always best to get skilled and qualified herbal advice during this process.

Withdrawal from Benzodiazepines

To successfully kick a benzodiazepine habit, it is essential that you know which type of benzodiazepine you are using. They can be divided into those that have active metabolites and therefore stay in the body longer, and those that spend less time in the body because they don't have such metabolites.

Drugs with a longer action include (the brand names are given in parentheses):

chlordiazepoxide (Librium)

diazepam (Valium)

flurazepam (Dalmane)

clorazepate (Tranxene)

Those with a shorter action include:

lorazepam (Ativan)

oxazepam (Serenid)

temazepam (Restoril)

This differentiation is important, not just for obvious therapeutic reasons but because the mode of withdrawal is different for each group. Withdrawal symptoms appear to be related to a rapid fall in blood levels of the drug, and it has been suggested that withdrawal is more severe and less successful in long-term users who are on a benzodiazepine with a shorter action.

First let's look at orthodox medicine's approach to withdrawal, followed by an herbal method.

Orthodox method

The orthodox approach to withdrawal is based on a gradual reduction of dosage with changes of drug at critical phases in the process. The following typical schedules do not take into account the effects of age, disease, or drug interactions on pharmacological activity.

People on shorter-action benzodiazepines might follow this withdrawal schedule:

1. Reduce the drug dosage by one-eighth every two to four weeks.

2. When the lowest therapeutic dosage is reached, change to the lowest dosage of a longer-action benzodiazepine.

People on longer-action benzodiazepines might follow this schedule:

1. Reduce the dosage by one-eighth every two to four weeks.

2. When the lowest therapeutic dosage is reached, further reduce the dosage every two weeks for four to eight weeks.

3. If physical symptoms arise, add Propranolol (60 to 120 mg daily) or Oxypertine (10 to 20 mg daily).

4. Stop taking benzodiazepines and reassess every four weeks.

Obviously, withdrawal by orthodox methods takes a long time. However, the whole process can be speeded up safely by simultaneously using herbal remedies. Not only will this reduce withdrawal symptoms but, more importantly, it will tone and strengthen the nervous system after its exposure to intense chemical stress, which was paradoxically meant to relieve the psychological impact of the stresses of daily life!

Herbal method

With the range of herbal remedies available to us, it is possible to ease the withdrawal process while treating specific bodily symptoms if they arise. It cannot be stressed enough that the aim here is to help people come off drugs and alleviate the need for artificial psychological support, not to replace benzodiazepines with herbal nervines.

Because the tranquilizers will have had a traumatic effect upon the whole system, the person's whole health and well-being must be attended to. The advice given here is for the nervous system itself, but the liver, kidneys, digestive tract, and so on must all be supported as well. Since each person's situation will be unique, this is where a qualified medical herbalist will be able to help. It is impossible to give general doses and specific prescriptions here. The herbs mentioned below should be studied in the herbal chapter of the book to find out which might be most appropriate in a particular case. However, the core of the process could be the following remedies:

Scullcap

Valerian

To these may be added other nervines, bitters, tonic herbs, and so on. Bitters will help the whole system regain vitality through a toning action on the digestive and endocrine systems.

Examples of bitters that might be used are:

Wormwood

Mugwort

The health of the liver must be supported because of its vital detoxifying role. Worth considering are:

Golden seal

Dandelion root

Any specific physical symptom can be treated with the appropriate herbs; for example:

Motherwort for heart palpitations

Comfrey or marshmallow root for stomach ulcers

It is difficult to generalize too freely, since different people will need different combinations of herbs to treat different combinations of symptoms, but remedies that I have found useful on occasions are:

Motherwort

Pasque flower

Oats

Lavender

St John's wort

Passionflower

This is just a partial list of my favorite remedies; for other herbalists, the list may well be different.

It is not possible to generalize about dosage levels and times either: taking a dose three times a day suits some people while taking the total daily dosage all at once helps others. A regular dose supplemented by extra doses when the person feels the need appears to be most effective. However, the dosage level is very variable, with some people being very sensitive to small doses of herbs such as scullcap, while others need much more.

The actual withdrawal procedure may be as follows:

1. For two to four days, take the benzodiazepine as usual, plus the herbs.

2. Reduce the drug dosage level by one-sixth, and take this dosage of the drug plus the herbs for the next four to five days.

3. Continue reducing the dosage level by one-sixth every four to five days. Increase the herbal-remedy dosages if needed, and take specific herbal remedies if help with any physical symptoms is needed.

This process can be accelerated or decelerated, as necessary. Do not try to go too fast, because if a feeling of failure develops, it compounds the whole process. Constant reassurance and support are vital, especially from close family members and work colleagues.

Supportive counseling and a willingness to gain insight from any psychological patterns that appear during the process helps. Sometimes active in-depth psychotherapy is useful, but should only be started if the person is feeling physically strong and able. Usually, there is more than enough going on at this time and it may be best to wait until the withdrawal process is complete.

Throughout the withdrawal process, a good, healthy, and balanced diet is essential, with a possible need for supplements of the B-complex vitamins and vitamin C.

ELEVEN

How to Prepare Herbal Remedies

There are a multitude of ways to prepare and use herbal remedies. Here, I will focus on the ways that aid the relaxation process most effectively. I won't explain the preparation of ointments, poultices, and suppositories, as they are rarely used for stress and tension relief. If you want to know more about them, any of the herbals mentioned in the bibliography will give recipes and instructions.

FRESH HERBS

It is almost always preferable to use freshly picked herbs, as they are rich in essential oils and still full of life. Of course, this is not always possible, in which case dried herbs or tinctures will do.

A few plants contain potentially dangerous natural chemicals that change to become quite safe when the plant is dried. An example of this kind of plant is pasque flower, which should never be used fresh but is perfectly safe when dried. Guidance about which herbs should not be used fresh is always given in herbals.

Some fresh herbs are delicious additions to our food, but if you choose to eat your medicine, these modern times necessitate careful field identification, as well as gathering in non-polluted places. For example, roadside dandelions do not make a healthy salad! It would be far better to combine a restful hike with the collection of a few wild plants. Have respect and be careful, not only to pick the right plant but also to pick only as much as you need.

Some fresh plants will yield their healing energy and constituents if you process them in a juicer, but you will need to drink the juice quickly or much of its energy will be oxidized and lost.

Infusions can be made with fresh herbs the same way as described below for dried herbs. Ensure that the teapot is covered so that a minimum of the essential aromatic oil escapes. If you can smell your fresh peppermint tea two rooms away, then most of its oil has been lost!

As a very rough guide, a handful of fresh leaves is equivalent to a teaspoon of dried herb. This approximation is useful, as most dosages are given for dried herbs or tinctures.

DRIED HERBS

A large variety of dried medicinal herbs is available these days. It is important to know that the cut, dried leaf is what the label says it is. As long as you buy dried herbs from a reputable company, you can be sure of their identity and quality.

The dosage for each herb varies. Details of specific levels is given in the last chapter, but since most of the remedies I am going to suggest in this book are quite safe, general guidelines can be followed without fear of overdose. However, always make sure you check the dosage level in an herbal before using an unfamiliar herb.

Teas

If the main ingredient of a remedy consists of leaves, petals, fruits, or even a root rich in aromatic oils, the tea should be made as an infusion. If it is woody, a root, bark, or a rhizome, then a decoction should be prepared.

Teas made in either of these ways will keep for three to four days if placed in a covered container in a refrigerator. If this is not possible, then they should be made fresh each day.

Infusions

Pour 1 pint of boiling water onto 1 ounce of finely chopped dried herb in a warmed pot. Cover and let steep for ten to fifteen minutes. Strain and keep in a covered container.

Decoctions

Add 1 ounce of chopped dried herb to 1 pint of cold water, bring to a boil, and gently simmer for ten to fifteen minutes. Let cool, strain, and keep in a covered container.

Dosage

Always check in an herbal that the dose you are taking is the correct one. For the vast majority of herbs, one wineglass (about 4 fluid ounces) of the infusion or decoction taken three times a day is safe. In most cases, a regular dose every eight hours is the most effective. The tea should usually be taken between meals.

Of course, a sleeping mixture is taken only at night, with the dosage depending upon your sensitivity to the herb. Experiment until you and the herb are familiar with each other, and the dosage is satisfactorily effective. This is quite safe!

Dosages should be reduced for the young and old. Up to the age of 10 and after the age of 70, only half the regular dosage should be taken.

Tinctures

An increasingly popular way of taking herbal remedies is in the form of a water/alcohol extract called a tincture. Tinctures are very concentrated and although they are easy to use for making medicines, the dosage calculations are very complex and they are best used under the guidance of a skilled medical herbalist.

Baths

A pleasant way to use relaxing herbs is in the form of a bath, where tea or tincture is added to hot bath water. A whole pint of an infusion or decoction is an appropriate amount to use for an adult.

Another way to prepare a bath would be to wrap the herbs in a muslin or cheesecloth bag and hang it under the hot-water faucet. When you run the water, it turns the bath into an infusion. Any herb can be used in this way, but the aromatic relaxing remedies are best.

Oils

Essential oils are used in quite different ways from other herbal remedies and are described in the section on aromatherapy. They make wonderful baths, too.

TWELVE

Herbs Used for Stress Control

T he herbs reviewed in this chapter by no means represent a complete list of herbal remedies that can be used in the treatment of stress-related problems. I have left out plants that are controlled substances or that are poisonous at certain dosage levels, as well as some of the less commonly used ones, such as asafoetida. Each of the herbs I have included is described in the same format, and includes a list of its "actions."

HERBAL ACTIONS

An action is one of the medical attributes of the herb, and it tells us how the plant may affect the body. Many different plants can have actions in common, and an understanding of these actions greatly aids the work of the medical herbalist. They can be explored further in some of the herbals suggested in the bibliography.

Some of the actions have rather outlandish names, so here is a partial list of definitions that covers some of the actions mentioned in this book:

ALTERNATIVE: Herbs that will gradually restore the proper functioning of the body and restore health. They are the old-fashioned "blood cleansers."

ANALGESIC ANODYNE: Pain relievers.

153

ANTICATARRHAL: Herbs that get rid of excess catarrh from the body.

ANTI-INFLAMMATORY: Remedies that reduce the inflammatory response in the body. They may be used internally or externally. These herbs are not suppressants in the way that steroid drugs may be.

ANTI-MICROBIAL: The anti-microbial herbs can help the body to destroy or resist pathogenic micro-organisms.

ANTISPASMODIC: The anti-spasmodics can prevent or ease spasms or cramps in the body.

AROMATIC: The aromatic herbs have a strong and often pleasant odor and can stimulate the digestive system. They are often used to add aroma and taste to other medicines.

ASTRINGENT: Astringents contract tissue by precipitating proteins and can thus reduce secretions and discharges. They contain tannins.

BITTER: Herbs that taste bitter act as stimulating tonics for the digestive system through a reflex via the taste buds.

CARDIAC TONIC: Cardiac tonics affect the heart. Their specific function should be looked up in the herbal section.

CARMINATIVE: The carminatives are rich in volatile oils and by their action stimulate the peristalsis of the digestive system and relax the stomach, thereby supporting the digestion and helping against gas in the digestive tract.

CHOLAGOGUE: The cholagogues stimulate the release and secretion of bile from the gallbladder, which can be a marked benefit in gallbladder problems. They also have a laxative effect on the digestive system since the amount of bile in the duodenum increases when one takes them.

DEMULCENT: Demulcents are rich in mucilage and can soothe and protect irritated or inflamed internal tissue.

DIAPHORETIC: Diaphoretics aid the skin in the elimination of toxins and promote perspiration.

DIURETIC: Diuretics increase the secretion and elimination of urine.

EMETIC: Emetics cause vomiting. Most of the herbs listed cause vomiting only when taken in high dosage.

EMMENAGOGUE: Emmenagogues stimulate and normalize menstrual flow. The term is also often used in the wider context of remedies that act as tonics to the female reproductive system.

EMOLLIENT: Emollients are applied to the skin to soften, soothe or protect it and act externally in a manner similar to the way demulcents act internally.

EXPECTORANT: Herbs that clear phlegm from the lungs.

HYPNOTIC: Herbs that induce sleep, not a hypnotic trance!

LAXATIVE: Herbs that promote bowel movements.

NERVINE: Remedies that affect the nervous system, usually toning and strengthening. Subcategories of this action are discussed in Chapter 5.

SEDATIVE: Plants that calm the nervous system, reducing anxiety and tension throughout the body. The herbal sedatives mentioned in this book are not addictive.

STIMULANT: These quicken and enliven the physiological functioning of the body. Using whole herbs usually gives optimum activity, rather than artificially inducing "hyped-up" activity as use of their chemical components in drug form may do.

TONIC: Herbs that strengthen and enliven either specific organs or the whole body.

VULNERARY: Plants that aid and speed the healing of cuts and wounds.

BETONY (WOOD BETONY)

Betonica officinalis (Stachys betonica), Labiatae

PART USED: Aerial parts.

COLLECTION: The aerial parts should be collected just before the flowers bloom. They should be dried carefully in the sun.

ACTIONS: Relaxant, sedative, a gentle stimulant of circulation to the head, nervine tonic, digestive bitter.

INDICATIONS: Betony feeds and strengthens the central nervous system while also having a sedative action upon the mind and "nerves" in general. It is used for nervous debility associated with anxiety and tension. It eases headaches and neuralgia when they are of nervous origin. Betony can help in sinus catarrh or other forms of catarrhal congestion in the head. Because of its bitter nature, it aids poor digestion due to debility.

COMBINATIONS: For the treatment of nervous headache, it combines with scullcap, lime blossom, and lavender flowers.

DOSAGE: 4 to 8 g (about 2 to 4 teaspoons) of the dried herb infused in 1 cup of water, three times a day.

BLACK COHOSH

Cimicifuga racemosa, Ranunculaceae

PART USED: Roots and rhizomes.

COLLECTION: The roots are unearthed with the rhizomes in autumn, after the fruits have ripened. They should be cut lengthwise and dried carefully.

ACTIONS: Emmenagogue, antispasmodic, alternative sedative, vasodilator, diaphoretic.

INDICATIONS: Black cohosh is a most valuable herb that comes to us via the North American Indians. It has a powerful action as a relaxant and as a normalizer of the female reproductive system, and so may be used beneficially in cases of painful or delayed menstruation. Ovarian cramps or cramping pain in the uterus are relieved by black cohosh. It has a normalizing action on the balance of female sex hormones and may safely be used to regain normal hormonal activity. It is very active in the treatment of rheumatic pains, but also in rheumatoid arthritis, in osteoarthritis, and in muscular and neurological pain. It can be used for sciatica and neuralgia. As a relaxing nervine, it may be used in many situations where such an agent is needed. Black cohosh reduces spasm and so aids in the treatment of pulmonary complaints such as whooping cough. It has been found beneficial in cases of tinnitus.

COMBINATIONS: For uterine conditions, combine with blue cohosh. For rheumatic problems, use with bogbean.

CAUTION: High doses of this plant may cause dizziness and agitation in sensitive people. It should not be used in pregnancy.

DOSAGE: 1 to 2 g (½–1 teaspoon) of the dried rhizome decocted in 1 cup of water as a tea, or its equivalent in tincture form, three times a day.

BLACK HAW

Viburnum prunifolium, Caprifoliaciae

PART USED: Bark of roots or stems.

COLLECTION: The bark from the roots and the trunk is collected in the autumn. The shrubs should be dug out and the bark stripped from the roots and trunk. The bark from the branches is collected in spring and summer. In both cases, the bark should be dried in the shade.

ACTIONS: Antispasmodic, sedative, hypotensive, astringent.

INDICATIONS: Black haw has a use very similar to cramp bark, to which it is closely related. It is a powerful relaxant of the uterus and is used for dysmenorrhea (uterine cramps or period pains) and false labor pains. It may also be used in threatened miscarriage. Its relaxant and sedative actions explain its power in reducing blood pressure, which happens through a relaxation of the peripheral blood vessels. Black haw also has a reputation in the treatment of vaginal and cervical discharges. It may be used as a general antispasmodic in the treatment of asthma.

COMBINATIONS: For threatened miscarriage, it combines well with false unicorn root and cramp bark.

DOSAGE: 4 to 8 g (2 to 4 teaspoons) of the dried bark decocted in 1 cup of water, three times a day as a tea, or as tincture.

BLACK HOREHOUND

Ballota nigra, Labiatae

PART USED: Aerial parts.

COLLECTION: The herb should be gathered just as it begins to bloom, and then dried.

ACTIONS: Antiemetic, sedative, mild astringent, emmenagogue, expectorant.

INDICATIONS: Black horehound – which should not be confused with white horehound – is an excellent remedy for the settling of nausea and vomiting where the cause lies within the nervous system rather than in the stomach. It may be used with safety in motion sickness, for example, where the nausea is triggered through the inner ear and the central nervous system. This herb will also be of value in helping the vomiting associated with pregnancy or nausea and vomiting due to nervousness. This remedy has a reputation as a normalizer of menstrual function and also as a mild expectorant.

COMBINATIONS: For the relief of nausea and vomiting, it may be combined with meadowsweet, chamomile, or peppermint.

DOSAGE: 2 to 4 g (1 to 2 teaspoons) of the dried herb infused in 1 cup of water as a tea or the equivalent in tincture form.

BLUE COHOSH

Caulophyllum thalictroides, Berberidaceae

PART USED: Roots and rhizomes.

COLLECTION: The roots and rhizomes are collected at the end of the growing season in the autumn, when they are richest in natural chemicals.

ACTIONS: Uterine tonic, emmenagogue, antispasmodic, antirheumatic.

INDICATIONS: Blue cohosh comes to us from the North American Indians, who called it squaw root and papoose root.

It is an excellent uterine and fallopian-tube tonic that may be used in any situation where there is a weakness or loss of tone. It may be used at any time during pregnancy if there is a threat of miscarriage. Similarly, because of its antispasmodic action, it will ease false labor pains. When labor begins, the use of blue cohosh just before birth helps ensure an easy delivery. In all these cases, it is a safe herb to use. As an emmenagogue, it can be used to bring on delayed or suppressed menstruation while ensuring that the pain that sometimes accompanies periods is relieved. It will alleviate the pains that may accompany any pelvic inflammation or even fibroids. Blue cohosh may be used in cases where an antispasmodic is needed, such as in colic, asthma, or nervous coughs. It has a reputation for easing rheumatic pain.

COMBINATIONS: To strengthen the uterus, it could be used with false unicorn root, motherwort, and yarrow.

DOSAGE: 1 to 2 g (½ to 1 teaspoon) of the dried rhizome decocted in 1 cup of water as a tea, or its equivalent in tincture form, three times a day.

BUGLEWEED

Lycopus europaeus, Labiatae

COMMON NAME: Water horehound.

PART USED: Aerial parts.

COLLECTION: The aerial parts should be collected just before the buds open, then dried.

ACTIONS: Cardioactive diuretic, peripheral vasoconstrictor, astringent, sedative, thyroxine antagonist, antitussive.

INDICATIONS: Bugleweed is a specific for overactive thyroid glands, especially where the symptoms include tightness of breathing, and palpitations that are of nervous origin. Bugleweed aids a weak heart where there is associated buildup of water in the body. As a sedative cough reliever, it eases irritating coughs, especially when they are of nervous origin. Such problems should, however, be diagnosed and treated by a qualified practitioner.

COMBINATIONS: Bugleweed may be used with nervines such as scullcap or valerian.

DOSAGE: 2 to 4 g (1 to 2 teaspoons) of the dried herb infused as a tea in 1 cup of water, or its equivalent in tincture form, 3 times a day.

CALIFORNIAN POPPY

Eschscholzia california, Papaveraceae

PART USED: Aerial parts.

COLLECTION: The aerial parts should be collected at the time of flowering, which is usually between June and September. They should be dried in the shade.

ACTIONS: Sedative, hypnotic, antispasmodic, anodyne.

INDICATIONS: Californian poppy has the reputation of being a nonaddictive alternative to the opium poppy, though it is less powerful. It has been used as a sedative and hypnotic for children, where there is overexcitability and sleeplessness. It can be used wherever an antispasmodic remedy is required. The American Indians used it for colic pains, and it may be useful in the treatment of gallbladder colic.

DOSAGE: 2 to 4 g (1–2 teaspoons) of the dried herb, infused as a tea, should be drunk at night to promote restful sleep.

CHAMOMILE, GERMAN

Matricaria chamomilla, Compositae

PART USED: Flowers.

COLLECTION: The flowers should be gathered between May and August when they are not wet with dew or rain. They should be dried with care at not too high a temperature.

ACTIONS: Relaxant, antispasmodic, carminative, anti-inflammatory, analgesic, antiseptic, vulnerary.

INDICATIONS: Chamomile is renowned for its medical and

household uses. The apparently endless list of conditions that it can help all fall into areas that the relaxing, carminative, and anti-inflammatory actions can aid. It is an excellent, gentle sedative, useful and safe for use with children. It will contribute its relaxing actions in any combinations and is thus used in anxiety and insomnia. Indigestion and inflammations such as gastritis are often eased with chamomile. Similarly, it can be used as a mouthwash for inflammations of the mouth such as gingivitis, and for bathing inflamed and sore eyes. As a gargle, it helps sore throats. As an inhalation over a steam bath, it speeds recovery from nasal catarrh. Externally, it speeds wound healing and reduces the swelling due to inflammation. As a carminative with relaxing properties, it eases flatulence and dyspeptic pain.

DOSAGE: 4 to 8 g (2 to 4 teaspoons) of the flower heads infused in 1 cup of water, or the equivalent in tincture form, three times a day or more. This tea can act as a wash for external use.

COWSLIP

Primula veris, Primulaceae

PART USED: Yellow petals and roots.

COLLECTION: The flower corollae should be gathered without the green calyx between March and May. Dry them quickly in the shade. The roots should be unearthed either before the plant flowers or in the autumn. Overcollecting has led to this beautiful plant becoming increasingly rare. Only pick if it is present in abundance and then only pick limited amounts.

ACTIONS: Flowers: sedative, antispasmodic; root: expectorant.

INDICATIONS: Cowslip is an excellent, generally applicable relaxing, sedative remedy. It eases reactions to stress and tension, relaxing nervous excitement and facilitating restful sleep. It may be used with safety in bronchitis, colds, chills, and congestive coughs. It has been used as part of a broad treatment for whooping cough. Try it for nervous headaches and insomnia.

COMBINATIONS: For stress-related problems, it may be used with any of the relaxing nervines, such as lime blossom or scullcap. For coughs, it may be used with coltsfoot, white horehound, and aniseed.

DOSAGE: 4 to 8 g (2 to 4 teaspoons) of the dried flowers infused in 1 cup of water, three times a day for anxiety or at night to aid sleep.

CRAMP BARK

Viburnum opulus, Caprifoliacea

PART USED: Bark.

COLLECTION: The bark is usually collected in April and May, cut into pieces, and dried.

ACTIONS: Antispasmodic, sedative, relaxant to smooth muscle, astringent.

INDICATIONS: Cramp bark indicates by its name the richly deserved reputation it has as a relaxer of muscular tension and spasm. It has two main areas of use: first, in muscular cramps, and second, in ovarian and uterine muscle problems. Cramp bark relaxes the uterus and so relieves painful cramps associated with periods (dysmenorrhea). In a similar way, it may be used to protect from threatened miscarriage. Cramp bark eases colicky pain in the intestines, gallbladder, and urinary system. Some cases of migraine and other conditions due to muscle spasm are eased. In conjunction with other remedies, it may help in the reduction of raised blood pressure. It has been used to help quiet overactive or convulsive states in children. Its astringent action gives it a role in the treatment of excessive blood loss in periods, and especially in bleeding associated with the menopause.

COMBINATIONS: For the relief of cramp, it may be combined with prickly ash and wild yam. For uterine and ovarian pains or threatened miscarriage, it may be used with black haw and valerian.

DOSAGE: 4 to 8 g (2–4 teaspoons) of the bark decocted in 1 cup of water, three times a day. The equivalent in tincture form can be used.

DAMIANA

Turnera aphrodisiaca, Turneraceae

PART USED: Leaves and stems.

COLLECTION: The leaves and stems are gathered at the time of flowering, and are then dried.

ACTIONS: Nerve tonic, antidepressant, urinary antiseptic, mild laxative.

INDICATIONS: Damiana is an excellent strengthening remedy for the nervous system. It has an ancient reputation as an aphrodisiac. While this may or may not be warranted, it has a definite tonic action on the central nervous and hormonal systems. The pharmacology of the plant suggests that its alkaloids could have a testosterone-like action (testosterone is a male hormone). As a useful antidepressant, damiana is considered to be a specific in cases of anxiety and depression where there is a sexual component. It may be used to strengthen the male sexual system.

COMBINATIONS: As a nerve tonic, it is often used with oats. Depending on the situation, it combines well with kola or scullcap.

DOSAGE: 3 to 6 g (about 1–2 teaspoons) of the herb infused in 1 cup of water, three times a day. The equivalent in tincture form can be used.

FEVERFEW

Tanacetum parthenium, Compositae

PART USED: Leaves.

COLLECTION: The leaves may be picked throughout the spring and summer, though just before flowering is best.

ACTIONS: Anti-inflammatory, vasodilatory, relaxant, digestive bitter, uterine stimulant.

INDICATIONS: Feverfew has regained its deserved reputation as a primary remedy in the treatment of migraine headaches, especially those that are relieved by applying warmth to the head. It may also help arthritis when it is in the painfully active, inflammatory stage. Dizziness and tinnitus may be eased, especially if feverfew is used in conjunction with other remedies. Painful periods and sluggish menstrual flow are also relieved by feverfew.

CAUTION: Feverfew should not be used during pregnancy because of stimulant action on the uterus. The fresh leaves may cause mouth ulcers in sensitive people.

DOSAGE: It is best to use the equivalent of one fresh leaf one to three times a day. Feverfew is best used fresh or frozen. Eat the leaf as a salad addition or on a sandwich. A 125 mg capsule of dried feverfew is the equivalent of a leaf.

GINSENG

Panax ginseng, Araliaceae

PART USED: Roots.

COLLECTION: Ginseng is cultivated in China, Korea, and in the northeastern region of the US (Panax quinquefolium).

ACTIONS: Antidepressant, increases resistance and improves both physical and mental performance, adaptogen.

INDICATIONS: Ginseng has an ancient history, and much folklore has accumulated about its actions and uses. Many of the claims that surround it are inflated, but it is clear that this is a unique plant. It has a direct action on the adrenal cortex, improving its responses to stress. Ginseng has the power to move people to their physical peak, and is especially helpful for debility, degenerative conditions, and problems of old age. In the short term, it improves stamina and concentration, aids healing, and generally increases resistance to stress. It raises lowered blood pressure to a normal level, and eases depression, especially where this is due to debility and exhaustion. It can be used for exhaustion states and weakness in general. It has a reputation as an aphrodisiac.

CAUTION: Ginseng should not be used over extensive periods of time, or if headaches start after using it. Avoid in conditions of high blood pressure.

DOSAGE: For treatment of debility or to aid the elderly, use 400 to 800 mg of the root a day. For short-term treatment of stress, use 600 to 2,000 mg of the dried root or its equivalent each day for up to three weeks.

See also Siberian Ginseng.

GOLDENROD

Solidago virgaurea, Compositae

PART USED: Aerial parts.

COLLECTION: The leaves and stems are picked in July and September just before flowering.

ACTIONS: Anti-inflammatory, anticatarrhal, urinary antiseptic, relaxant.

INDICATIONS: While primarily used as an excellent herb for relieving upper respiratory catarrh, it also helps where such problems are compounded by nervous tension and restlessness.

DOSAGE: 4 to 8 g (about 2–4 teaspoons) of the dried herb infused in 1 cup of water, three times a day.

GOTU KOLA

Hydrocotyle asiatica, Umbelliferae

PART USED: Leaves and stems.

ACTIONS: Relaxant, nervine tonic, digestive bitter, diuretic, anti-inflammatory, vulnerary.

INDICATIONS: This tropical plant has a growing reputation as a restorative, relaxing remedy for the nervous system. It may be of help in a whole range of neurological and mental disturbances, especially stress-related debility. It may be used in inflammatory diseases such as rheumatism. In the East, gotu kola has a good reputation for the treatment of poorly healing wounds and ulcers.

DOSAGE: 0.5 to 2 g (about 1 teaspoon) of the dried herb infused in 1 cup of water, three times a day.

HOPS

Humulus lupulus, Cannabinaceae

PART USED: Flower inflorescences.

COLLECTION: The hops cones are gathered before they are fully ripe, usually in August and September. They should be dried with care in the shade.

ACTIONS: Sedative, hypnotic, antiseptic, astringent, bitter.

INDICATIONS: Hops is a remedy that has a marked relaxing effect upon the central nervous system. It is used extensively for the treatment of insomnia. It eases tension and anxiety, and may be used where tension leads to restlessness, headache, and possibly indigestion. As an astringent with these relaxing properties, it can be used in conditions such as mucous colitis. It should, however, be avoided where there is a marked degree of depression, as this may be accentuated. Externally, the antiseptic action is utilized for the treatment of ulcers.

COMBINATIONS: For insomnia, it can be combined with valerian and passionflower.

CAUTION: Do not use in cases with marked depression.

DOSAGE: 0.5 to 1 g (about 1 teaspoon) of the flowers as an infused tea three times a day. A much stronger tea may be used at night to promote sleep.

HYSSOP

Hyssopus officinalis, Labiatae

PART USED: Aerial parts.

COLLECTION: The flowering tops of the plant should be collected in August and dried in the sun.

ACTIONS: Antispasmodic, expectorant, diaphoretic, sedative, carminative.

INDICATIONS: Hyssop has an interesting range of uses that are largely attributable to the antispasmodic action of the volatile oil. It is used in coughs, bronchitis, and chronic catarrh. Its diaphoretic properties explain its use in the common cold. As a nervine, it may be used in anxiety states, hysteria, and petit mal (a form of epilepsy).

COMBINATIONS: It may be combined with white horehound and coltsfoot in the treatment of coughs and bronchitis. For the common cold, it may be mixed with boneset, elder flower, and peppermint.

DOSAGE: 4 to 8 g (2 to 4 teaspoons) of the dried herb infused in 1 cup of water, three times a day.

JAMAICA DOGWOOD

Piscidia erythrina, Leguminosae

PART USED: Stem bark.

COLLECTION: The bark is collected in vertical strips from trees growing in the Caribbean, Mexico, and Texas.

ACTIONS: Sedative, anodyne.

INDICATIONS: Jamaica dogwood is a powerful sedative, used in its West Indian homeland as a fish poison. While not being poisonous to humans, the given dosage level should not be exceeded. It is a powerful remedy for the treatment of painful conditions such as neuralgia and migraine. It can also be used in the relief of ovarian and uterine pain. Perhaps its main use is in insomnia that is related to nervous tension or pain. It may be helpful in some cases of migraine.

COMBINATIONS: For the easing of insomnia, it is best combined with hops and valerian. For dysmenorrhea (painful periods), it may be used with black haw.

DOSAGE: 0.5 to 2 g (1 teaspoon) of the dried bark decocted in 1 cup of water as a tea, three times a day. The equivalent in tincture form can be used as well.

KAVA KAVA

Piper methysticum, Piperaceae

PART USED: Rhizomes.

ACTIONS: Urinary antiseptic and diuretic, circulatory stimulant, antispasmodic, psychoactive.

INDICATIONS: This exotic herb from the South Pacific has its main use in the treatment of urinary infection. It can be used in small dosage as a mental stimulant, but at higher dosage it will slow down mental awareness. In its native lands, the fresh plant has been used to produce an active psychedelic product.

DOSAGE: 1 to 4 g (1–1½ teaspoons) of the rhizome decocted in 1 cup of water, three times a day.

KOLA

Cola vera, Sterculiaceae

PART USED: Seed kernels.

COLLECTION: The kola tree grows in tropical Africa and is also cultivated in South America. The seeds are collected when ripe and are initially white, turning a characteristic red upon drying.

ACTIONS: Stimulant to the central nervous system, antidepressant, astringent, diuretic.

INDICATIONS: Kola has a marked stimulating effect on human consciousness. It can be used wherever there is a need for direct stimulation, which is less often than is usually thought. With proper health and therefore right functioning, the nervous system does not need such help. In the short term, it may be used for nervous debility, in states of atony and weakness. It can act as a specific in nervous diarrhea. It aids in states of depression and may in some people give rise to euphoric states. In some varieties of migraine, it can help greatly. Through stimulation, it can be a valuable part of the treatment for anorexia. It can be viewed as specific in cases of depression associated with weakness and debility.

COMBINATIONS: Kola will go well with oats, damiana, and scullcap.

DOSAGE: 2 to 4 g (1 to 2 teaspoons) of the powdered seeds three times a day. The equivalent tincture form can be used.

LADY'S SLIPPER

Cypripripedium pubescens, Orchidaceae

PART USED: Roots.

COLLECTION: Lady's slipper is a protected plant in the United Kingdom and so should never be collected if found wild.

ACTIONS: Sedative, hypnotic, antispasmodic, nervine tonic.

INDICATIONS: Lady's slipper is one of the most widely applicable nervines available to us. It may be used in all stress reactions, emotional tension, and anxiety states. It helps elevate the mood, especially where depression is present. It can help in easing nervous pain, though it is best used in combination with other herbs for this purpose. It is perhaps at its best when treating anxiety that is associated with insomnia.

COMBINATIONS: It combines well with oats and scullcap. For nerve pain, it may be used with Jamaica dogwood, passionflower, and valerian.

DOSAGE: 2 to 8 g (1–4 teaspoons) of the dried root infused in 1 cup of water, three times a day. A stronger tea can be drunk at night. This root is made into an infusion rather than a decoction because it is so rich in volatile oil. The equivalent in tincture form can be used.

LAVENDER

Lavendula officinalis, Labiatae

PART USED: Flowers.

COLLECTION: The flowers should be gathered just before opening between June and September. They should be dried gently at a temperature not above 35 degrees C.

ACTIONS: Carminative, antispasmodic, antidepressant, rubefacient.

INDICATIONS: This beautiful herb has many uses – culinary, cosmetic, and medicinal. It is an effective herb for headaches, especially when they are related to stress. Lavender can be quite effective in the raising of depression, especially if used in conjunction with other remedies. As a gentle strengthening tonic of the nervous system, it may be used in states of nervous debility and exhaustion. It can be used to soothe and promote natural sleep. Because of its carminative oil, lavender eases digestive colic and flatulent dyspepsia. Externally, the oil is used as a stimulating liniment to help ease the aches and pains of rheumatism and migraine.

COMBINATIONS: For depression, it combines well with rosemary, kola, damiana, or scullcap. For headaches, it may be used with lady's slipper or valerian.

DOSAGE: An infusion of fresh or dried flowers is made with 4 to 8 g (2 to 4 teaspoons) per cup of water, taking care to cover the pot so that the aroma is not lost. Take three times a day.

LEMON BALM

Melissa officinalis, Labiatae

PART USED: Aerial parts.

COLLECTION: The plant should be collected just before the flower blossoms open in midsummer. They should be collected on a dry day and dried carefully in the shade.

ACTIONS: Relaxant, carminative.

INDICATIONS: This herb can be used with equal value for tension affecting the nervous system and digestive system. It is widely applicable for all varieties of anxiety- and tension-related problems. It has particular relevance for childhood problems such as overactivity. It will ease many indigestion symptoms. It has been used in high dosage to treat shingles.

DOSAGE: 4 to 8 g (2 to 4 teaspoons) of the dried herb, infused in 1 cup of water, three times a day, or as required.

LIFE ROOT

Senecio aureus, Compositae

PART USED: Aerial parts.

COLLECTION: Pick just before the small flowers open in the summer.

ACTIONS: Uterine relaxant and tonic, relaxant.

INDICATIONS: A wonderful remedy for gynecological conditions, especially menopausal problems. Almost a specific for the emotional upsets of menopause.

CAUTION: This herb should not be used during pregnancy.

DOSAGE: 2 to 4 g (1 to 2 teaspoons) of the dried herb, infused in 1 cup of water, three times a day.

LIME BLOSSOM (LINDEN)

Tilia europaea, Tiliaceae

PART USED: Flowers.

COLLECTION: The flowers should be gathered immediately after flowering in midsummer. They should be collected on a dry day and dried carefully in the shade.

ACTIONS: Nervine, antispasmodic, diaphoretic, diuretic, mild astringent.

INDICATIONS: Lime blossom is well known as a relaxing

remedy for use in nervous tension. It has a reputation as a prophylactic against the development of arteriosclerosis and hypertension. It is considered a specific in the treatment of raised blood pressure associated with arteriosclerosis and nervous tension. Its relaxing action combined with a general effect upon the circulatory system give lime blossom a role in the treatment of some forms of migraine. Its diaphoretic action combined with its relaxant action explain its value in feverish colds and flu.

COMBINATIONS: In raised blood pressure, it may be used with hawthorn and mistletoe; in nervous tension, with hops; and in the common cold, with elder flower.

DOSAGE: 4 to 8 g (2 to 4 teaspoons) of the dried flowers, infused in 1 cup of water, three times a day. A stronger tea may be used at night.

LOBELIA

Lobelia inflata, Campanulaceae

PART USED: Aerial parts.

COLLECTION: The entire plant above ground should be collected at the end of flowering time, usually between August and September. The seed pods should be collected as well.

ACTIONS: Respiratory stimulant, antiasthmatic, antispasmodic, expectorant, emetic.

INDICATIONS: Lobelia is one of the most useful systemic relaxants available to us. It has a general depressant action on the central and autonomic nervous systems and on neuromuscular action. It may be used in many conditions in combination with other herbs, to further their effectiveness if relaxation is needed. Its primary specific use is in bronchitic asthma and bronchitis. An analysis of the action of its alkaloids reveals apparently paradoxical effects. Lobeline is a powerful respiratory stimulant, while isolobinine is an emetic and respiratory relaxant, which stimulates catarrhal secretion and expectoration while relaxing the muscles of the respiratory system. The overall action is a truly holistic combination of stimulation and relaxation! It plays a role in the holistic treatment of allergic, inflammatory, and hypersensitivity reactions. It can be used externally to ease muscle spasms.

COMBINATIONS: It combines well with cayenne, grindelia, pill-bearing spurge, sundew, and ephedra in the treatment of asthma.

DOSAGE: As a dried herb, this remedy should be used under the supervision of a qualified herbalist.

MATE

Ilex paraguariensis, Aquifoliaceae

PART USED: Leaves.

ACTIONS: Central nervous system stimulant, antispasmodic, diuretic.

INDICATIONS: Mate is used in South America in the way tea is used in Britain. Medically, it helps with nervous headaches associated with fatigue. It may help control excessive appetite (if you're lucky!).

CAUTION: As with other caffeine-rich herbs such as tea and coffee, mate should be drunk in moderation.

DOSAGE: 2 to 4 g (1 teaspoon) of the dried leaves infused in 1 cup of water, drunk when wanted.

MISTLETOE

Viscum album, Lorantheaceae

PART USED: Leafy twigs.

COLLECTION: The young leafy twigs should be collected in the spring.

ACTIONS: Nervine, hypotensive, cardiac depressant, possible antitumor.

INDICATIONS: Mistletoe is an excellent relaxing nervine indicated in many cases. It quietens, soothes, and tones the nervous system. This remedy acts directly on the vagus nerve to reduce the heart rate while strengthening the wall of the peripheral capillaries. It thus acts to reduce blood pressure and ease arteriosclerosis. Where there is nervous quickening of the heart (nervous tachycardia), it may be very helpful. Headache due to high blood pressure is relieved by it. It has been shown by current cancer research to have some antitumor activity.

COMBINATIONS: It combines well with hawthorn berries and lime blossom in the treatment of raised blood pressure.

CAUTION: Do not use mistletoe berries!

DOSAGE: 1 to 2 g (½–1 teaspoon) of the dried leaves infused in 1 cup of water, up to three times a day.

MOTHERWORT

Leonurus cardiaca, Labiatae

PART USED: Aerial parts.

COLLECTION: The stalks should be gathered at the time of flowering, which is usually between June and September.

ACTIONS: Sedative, emmenagogue, antispasmodic, uterine tonic, cardiac tonic, carminative.

INDICATIONS: The names of this plant show its range of uses: motherwort shows its relevance to menstrual and uterine conditions while cardiaca indicates its use in heart and circulation treatments. It is valuable in the stimulation of delayed or suppressed menstruation, especially where there is anxiety or tension involved. It is a useful relaxing tonic for aiding in menopausal changes. It may be used to ease false labor pains. Disturbance of menstrual cycles due to tension and worry are also eased by this herb. It is an excellent tonic for the heart, strengthening without straining. It is a specific for over-rapid heartbeat brought about by anxiety and other such causes. It may be used in all heart conditions that are associated with anxiety and tension.

DOSAGE: 4 to 8 g (2 to 4 teaspoons) of the dried herb infused in 1 cup of water, or the equivalent in tincture form.

MUGWORT

Artemisia vulgaris, Compositae

PART USED: Leaves or roots.

COLLECTION: The leaves and flowering stalks should be gathered just at blossoming time, which is usually between July and September.

ACTIONS: Bitter tonic, stimulant, nervine tonic, emmenagogue.

INDICATIONS: Mugwort can be used wherever a digestive stimulant is called for. It aids the digestion through the bitter stimulation of the digestive juices, while also providing a carminative oil. It has a mildly nervine action in aiding depression and easing tension, which appears to be due to the volatile oil it contains, so it is essential that this oil not be lost in preparation. Mugwort can also be used as an emmenagogue to aid normal menstrual flow.

DOSAGE: 2 to 4 g (1 teaspoon) of the dried herb, infused in 1 cup of water, three times a day. The equivalent in tincture form can be used.

OATS

Avena sativa, Gramineae

PART USED: Grains and straw.

COLLECTION: Oats are usually harvested in August. The stalks are cut, bound together, and left upright to dry. Then the grain is threshed out. The crushed dry stalks can be used as straw.

ACTIONS: Nervine tonic, antidepressant, nutritive, demulcent, vulnerary.

INDICATIONS: Oats is one of the best remedies for "feeding" the nervous system, especially when under stress. It is considered a specific in cases of nervous debility and exhaustion when associated with depression. It may be used with most of the other nervines, both relaxant and stimulant, to strengthen the whole of the nervous system. It is also used in general debility. The high levels of silicic acid in the straw explain its use as a remedy for skin conditions, especially in external applications.

COMBINATIONS: For depression, it may be used with scullcap and lady's slipper.

CAUTION: Should not be used by people who have gluten allergies.

DOSAGE: 4 to 8 g (2–4 teaspoons) of the grain or oatmeal infused in 1 cup of water, three times a day. Cooked oatmeal provides a good source.

PASQUE FLOWER

Anemone pulsatilla, Ranunculaceae

PART USED: Aerial parts.

COLLECTION: The stalks should be gathered at the time of flowering, which is usually in March or April.

ACTIONS: Sedative, analgesic, antispasmodic, antibacterial.

INDICATIONS: Pasque flower is an excellent relaxing nervine for use in problems relating to nervous tension and spasm in the reproductive system. It may be used with safety in the relief of painful periods (dysmenorrhea), ovarian pain, and painful conditions of the testes. Pasque flower has valuable properties in easing premenstrual tension and anxiety associated with menopause. It may be used to reduce tension reactions and the headaches associated with them. It helps in insomnia and general overactivity. Its antibacterial actions give this herb a role in treating infections that affect the skin, especially boils. It is similarly useful in the treatment of respiratory infections and asthma. The oil or tincture eases earache.

COMBINATIONS: For painful periods, it combines well with cramp bark. For skin conditions, it combines with echinacea.

CAUTION: Do not use the fresh plant!

DOSAGE: 1 to 2 g (½ to 1 teaspoon) of the dried leaves infused in 1 cup of water, three times a day.

PASSIONFLOWER

Passiflora incarnata, Passifloraceae

PART USED: Leaves.

COLLECTION: If the foliage alone is to be collected, this should happen just before the flowers bloom, usually between May and July. The foliage may be collected with the fruit after flowering. It should be dried in the shade.

ACTIONS: Sedative, hypnotic, antispasmodic, anodyne.

INDICATIONS: Passionflower is the herb of choice for treating intransigent insomnia. It aids the transition into a restful sleep without any "narcotic" hangover. It may be used wherever an antispasmodic is required; for example, in Parkinson's disease, seizures, and hysteria. It can be very effective in nerve pain such as neuralgia and in the viral infection of the nerves called shingles. It may be used in asthma where there is much spasmodic activity, especially when there is associated tension.

COMBINATIONS: For insomnia, it combines well with valerian, hops, and Jamaica dogwood.

DOSAGE: 0.5 to 1 g (½ teaspoon) infused in 1 cup of water, three times a day. For use at night, make a much stronger tea.

PEPPERMINT

Mentha piperita, Labiatae

PART USED: Aerial parts.

COLLECTION: The aerial parts are collected just before the flowers open.

ACTIONS: Carminative, antispasmodic, aromatic, diaphoretic, antiemetic, nervine, antiseptic, analgesic.

INDICATIONS: Peppermint is one of the best carminative

agents available. It has a relaxing effect on the visceral muscles, has antiflatulent properties, and stimulates bile and digestive juice secretion, all of which help to explain its value in relieving intestinal colic, flatulent dyspepsia, and other associated conditions. The volatile oil acts as a mild anesthetic to the stomach wall, which allays feelings of nausea and the desire to vomit. It helps relieve the vomiting associated with pregnancy and travel sickness. Peppermint plays a role in the treatment of ulcerative colitis and Crohn's disease. Peppermint is most valuable in the treatment of fevers and especially in colds and influenza. As an inhalant, it can be used as a temporary treatment of nasal catarrh. Where migraine headaches are associated with digestion, this herb may be used. As a nervine, it acts as a tonic, easing anxiety, tension, hysteria, and so on. In painful periods (dysmenorrhea), it relieves the pain and eases associated tension. Externally, it may be used to relieve itching and inflammations.

COMBINATIONS: For colds and influenza, it may be used with boneset, elder flowers, and yarrow.

DOSAGE: 4 to 8 g (2 to 4 teaspoons) of the dried leaves infused in 1 cup of water, three times a day.

ROSEMARY

Rosemarinus officinalis, Labiatae

PART USED: Leaves and twigs.

COLLECTION: The leaves may be gathered throughout the summer but are at their best during flowering time.

ACTIONS: Carminative, aromatic, antispasmodic, antidepressant, antiseptic, rubefacient, parasiticide.

INDICATIONS: Rosemary acts as a circulatory and nervine stimulant, which, in addition to its toning and calming effect on the digestion, makes it a remedy that is used where psychological tension is present. This may appear as, for example, flatulent dyspepsia, headache, or depression associated with debility. It may be of use in migraine, palpitations, and other signs of nervous tension. Externally, it may be used to ease muscular pain, sciatica, and neuralgia. It acts as a stimulant to the hair follicles and may be used in premature baldness; the oil is most effective here.

COMBINATIONS: For depression, it may be used with scullcap, kola, and oats.

DOSAGE: 4 to 8 g (2 to 4 teaspoons) of the dried herb infused in 1 cup of water, three times a day. It is most effective when used over a period of at least three weeks.

ST. JOHN'S WORT

Hypericum perforatum, Hypericaceae

PART USED: Aerial parts.

COLLECTION: The entire plant above ground should be collected when in flower and dried as quickly as possible.

ACTIONS: Nervine tonic, astringent, local anodyne.

INDICATIONS: Taken internally, St. John's wort has a sedative and pain-reducing effect, which gives it a place in the treatment of neuralgia, anxiety, tension, and similar problems. Where these problems have been going on long enough to produce debility and fatigue, St. John's wort will prove invaluable. It is especially useful when menopausal changes trigger irritability and anxiety. It is recommended, however, that it not be used when there is marked depression. In addition to neuralgic pain, it eases fibrositis, sciatica, and rheumatic pain. Externally, it is a valuable healing and anti-inflammatory remedy. As a lotion, it speeds the healing of wounds and bruises, varicose veins, and mild burns. The oil is especially useful for the healing of sunburn, neuralgia, and fibrositis.

DOSAGE: 4 to 8 g (2 to 4 teaspoons) infused in 1 cup of water, three times a day. The tincture has all the value of the dried plant. This is another herb that achieves best results when used over a period of time.

SCULLCAP

Scutellaria laterifolia, Labiatae

PART USED: Aerial parts.

COLLECTION: The whole of the aerial parts should be collected late in the flowering period, usually during August and September.

ACTIONS: Nervine tonic, sedative, antispasmodic.

INDICATIONS: Scullcap is perhaps the most widely relevant nervine available to us. It relaxes nervous tension and anxiety, while at the same time renewing and revitalizing the central nervous system. It has a specific use in the treatment of seizures and hysterical states, as well as epilepsy. It may be used in all exhausted, debilitated, or depressed conditions. It can be used with complete safety in the easing of premenstrual tension.

COMBINATIONS: It combines well with valerian.

DOSAGE: 4 to 8 g (2–4 teaspoons) infused in 1 cup of water, three times a day. The tincture is of similar value.

SIBERIAN GINSENG

Eleutherococcus senticosus, Araliaceae

PART USED: Roots.

ACTIONS: Adaptogen, circulatory stimulant, vasodilator; similar in action to the Asiatic Ginseng.

INDICATIONS: A valuable remedy for improving stamina when the person is under excessive physical and mental demands. It improves vitality in the face of exhaustion, debility, and depression. It appears to promote an increase in resistance to more generalized stresses, such as infections, disease, and aging. There is some evidence that it can reverse the early stages of arteriosclerosis.

DOSAGE: 2 to 4 g (1–2 teaspoons) of the root decocted in 1 cup of water, three times a day.

SQUAW VINE

Mitchelia repens, Rubiaceae

PART USED: Aerial parts.

ACTIONS: Nervine tonic, uterine tonic.

INDICATIONS: While primarily useful in facilitating labor and easing delivery, squaw vine is an excellent remedy for painful periods, nervous debility, exhaustion, and general irritability.

DOSAGE: 4 to 8 g (2 to 4 teaspoons) of the dried herb infused in 1 cup of water, three times a day.

SWEET FLAG

Acorus calamus, Araceae

PART USED: Rhizomes.

ACTION: Carminative, relaxant.

INDICATIONS: Specific for overacidity of the stomach and peptic ulceration. As a relaxing nervine with marked carminative properties, it eases intestinal colic and flatulence.

DOSAGE: 2 to 4 g (1–2 teaspoons) of the rhizome decocted in 1 cup of water, three times a day.

VALERIAN

Valeriana officinalis, Valerianaceae

PART USED: Rhizomes and roots.

COLLECTIONS: The roots should be unearthed in late autumn, cleaned thoroughly, and dried in the shade.

ACTIONS: Sedative, hypnotic, antispasmodic, hypotensive, carminative.

INDICATIONS: Valerian is one of the most useful relaxing nervines that is available to us. This fact is recognized by orthodox medicine, as is shown by its inclusion in many pharmacopeias as a sedative. It may safely be used to reduce tension and anxiety, overexcitability, and hysterical states. It is an effective aid in insomnia, producing a natural, healing sleep. As an antispasmodic herb, it aids in the relief of cramp and intestinal colic, and is also useful for the cramps and pain of periods. As a pain reliever, it is most indicated where pain is associated with tension. Valerian can help in migraine and rheumatic pain.

COMBINATIONS: For the relief of tension, it combines most effectively with scullcap. For insomnia, it can be combined with passionflower and hops. For the treatment of cramps, it works well with cramp bark.

DOSAGE: 2 to 8 g (1 to 4 teaspoons) of the dried root infused in 1 cup of water, three times a day. This root is used as an infusion because of its rich volatile oil content.

VERVAIN

Verbena officinalis, Labiatae

PART USED: Aerial parts.

COLLECTION: The herb should be collected just before the flowers open, usually in July, and dried quickly.

ACTIONS: Nervine tonic, sedative, antispasmodic, diaphoretic, possible galactagogue, hepatic.

INDICATIONS: Vervain strengthens the nervous system while relaxing tension. It can be used to ease depression and melancholia, especially when this follows illnesses such as influenza. Vervain may be used to help in seizures and hysteria. As a diaphoretic, it can be used in the early stages of fevers. As a hepatic remedy, it is helpful in inflammation of the gallbladder and jaundice. It may be used as a mouthwash against caries and gum disease.

COMBINATIONS: In the treatment of depression, it may be used with scullcap, oats, and lady's slipper.

DOSAGE: 4 to 8 g (2 to 4 teaspoons) infused in 1 cup of water, three times a day.

WILD LETTUCE

Lactuca virosa, Compositae

PART USED: Leaves.

COLLECTION: The leaves should be gathered in June and July, and then dried.

ACTIONS: Sedative, anodyne, hypnotic.

INDICATIONS: The latex of wild lettuce was at one time sold as "lettuce opium," reflecting the use of this herb! It is a valuable remedy for use in insomnia, restlessness, excitability (especially in children), and other manifestations of an overactive nervous system. As an antispasmodic, it can be used as part of the holistic treatment of whooping cough and of dry, irritated coughs in general. It relieves colic pains in the intestines and uterus, and so may be used for painful periods. It eases muscular pains related to rheumatism. It has also been used as an aphrodisiac.

COMBINATIONS: For irritable coughs, it may be used with wild cherry bark. For insomnia, it combines well with valerian and pasque flower.

DOSAGE: 2 to 4 g (1 to 2 teaspoons) of the dried herb infused in 1 cup of water, three times a day, or as a stronger tea at night.

WORMWOOD

Artemisia absinthium, Compositae

PART USED: Leaves and flowering tops.

COLLECTION: The leaves and flowering tops are gathered at the end of the flowering period, usually between July and September.

ACTIONS: Bitter tonic, carminative, anthelmintic, anti-inflammatory.

INDICATIONS: Traditionally, wormwood has been used in a wide range of conditions. The validity of most of these uses has been verified by analysis of the herb. It is primarily used as a bitter and therefore has the effect of stimulating and invigorating the whole digestive process. It may be used where there is indigestion, especially when due to a deficient quantity or quality of gastric juice. It is a powerful remedy in the treatment of worm infestations, particularly roundworm and pinworm. It may also be used to help the body deal with fever and infections. Due to its general tonic action, it is useful for many diverse conditions because it benefits the body in general.

DOSAGE: 1 to 2 g (1 teaspoon) of the dried herb drunk as an infused tea three times a day, or the equivalent in tincture form.

Selected Bibliography

HERBALS

British Herbal Medicine Association, *British Herbal Pharmacopoeia,* Volumes 1, 2, and 3

Ceres, *The Healing Power of Herbal Teas,* Thorsons Publishers, Inc. (1985)

Christopher, John R., *School of Natural Healing,* BiWorld (1976)

Grieve, M., *A Modern Herbal,* Dover Publications (1931)

Hoffmann, David L., *The Holistic Herbal,* Findhorn (1983)

Lust, John, *The Herb Book,* Bantam Books (1974)

Mills, Simon Y., *The Dictionary of Modern Herbalism,* Thorsons Publishers, Inc. (1985)

Parvati, Jeannine, *Hygieia,* Wildwood House (1978)

Potter's New Cyclopaedia of Botanical Drugs, Health Science Press (1975)

Priest & Priest, *Herbal Medication,* Fowler (1982)

Tierra, Michael, The Way of Herbs (1983)

GENERAL BOOKS OF HELP AND ADVICE

Benson, Herbert, *Relaxation Response,* Avon Books (1976)

Chaitow, Leon, *Your Complete Stress-Proofing Program,* Thorsons Publishers, Inc. (1985)

Cox, Tom, *Stress,* Macmillan Press (1983)

Davis, Martha; McKay, Matthew; and Robbins Eshelman, Elizabeth, *The Relaxation and Stress Reduction Workbook,* New Harbinger (1985)

Horn, Sandra, *Relaxation: Modern Techniques for Stress Management,* Thorsons Publishers, Inc. (1986)

LeShan, Lawrence, *Holistic Health,* Turnstone Press (1982)

Rowe, Dorothy, *Depression—A Way Out of Your Prison,* Routledge & Kegan Paul (1983)

Shuttle, Penelope and Redgrove, Peter, *The Wise Wound, Eve's Curse and Every Woman,* Gallancz (1978)

Simonton, Carl and Stephanie, *Getting Well Again,* Tarcher (1978)

Which? Magazine, *Living with Stress,* Consumer's Association (1982)

Index